IMMUNISATION

IMMUNISATION

George Dick

MD, D.SC, MPH, FRCP, FRC.PATH, FIMLT

Assistant Director of the British Postgraduate
Medical Federation; Regional Postgraduate Dean
to the Southwest Thames Regional Health
Authority, England; Honorary Consultant at the
Institute of Child Health, London; Professor
of Pathology at London University

UPDATE BOOKS
LONDON/NEW JERSEY

Published by
UPDATE PUBLICATIONS LTD

Available in the United Kingdom and Eire in paperback edition from
Update Publications Ltd
33/34 Alfred Place
London WC1E 7DP
England

Available outside the United Kingdom in hardback edition from
Update International Inc.
2337 Lemoine Avenue
Fort Lee
New Jersey 07024
USA

First published 1978
ISBN 978-0-906141-03-8   ISBN 978-94-011-7633-0 (eBook)
DOI 10.1007/978-94-011-7633-0

British Library Cataloguing in Publication Data
Dick, George
Immunisation.
1. Immunisation
I. Title
614.4'7   RA638
ISBN 978-0-906141-03-8

Contents

Preface

The development of immunisation has been one of the most striking features in the control of infectious disease in the twentieth century. This book takes into account the need for a simple, concise account of immunisation procedures not only in the UK and USA but also in other countries, and to this end a special chapter on immunisation in developing countries has been included. Following two introductory chapters, there are nine chapters on various diseases and the vaccines that have been developed to combat them. In each of these chapters, a short discussion of the epidemiology of the disease and the history of immunisation against it is followed by a description of the vaccine, its efficacy, contraindications to its use and future developments. The book concludes with four general chapters on vaccines for travel, vaccines for selective use, passive immunisation and immunisation in tropical environments.

The demand for this book follows the popularity of a series of articles on immunisation which appeared in *Update*. These have been expanded and largely rewritten. I have drawn on many expert sources and have made an effort to provide a balanced and non-controversial opinion with a discussion of alternative procedures where indicated.

Immunisation is intended not only for the family practitioner but also for many specialists, particularly paediatricians, community physicians, Armed Forces medical officers, and all those concerned with immigration procedures and with the spread of infectious diseases. Medical students, nurses and paramedical staff will also find much of value.

George Dick
London

1. Introduction

The prevention of infectious diseases depends on controlling or eliminating the source of infection, breaking the chain of transmission or increasing the resistance of the individual to infection by general means or by immunisation.

Many infectious diseases can be prevented without immunisation, because once the natural history of the disease is understood, the source may be eliminated or transmission prevented. Thus, the prevention of rabies in the United Kingdom depends on controlling the importation of dogs and other animals from countries with endemic rabies (which now includes much of Europe). Similarly, psittacosis is prevented in man, not by routine immunisation but by the control of imported parrots. When it was discovered in the 19th century that cholera and typhoid epidemics were regularly transmitted by faecal contamination of water, the provision of clean water supplies nearly eradicated these diseases from many countries without recourse to immunisation. Again, yellow fever in urban areas was eliminated at the beginning of this century when it was discovered that it was transmitted by *Aedes aegypti*. All that was required was to stop the breeding of that particular mosquito.

Socioeconomic Conditions

The great reduction, and in some cases the virtual disappearance, of many diseases in some countries has been partly due to improved social conditions resulting in increased resistance to infection and reduction in transmission. Thus the mortality from measles in England at the beginning of this century was 30 per 100,000. In 1965, before the introduction of any vaccine, it had fallen to 0.1 per 100,000. Today the mortality of measles in many developing countries is of the same order as it was in Britain at the turn of the century.

Immunisation

In addition to the changes in incidence and mortality of some diseases which have apparently been brought about by changes in living conditions, there are other unknown factors which have affected the ecology of some diseases. Thus, scarlet fever was a mild disease when it was described by Sydenham in 1675, but in the middle of the 18th century it caused many deaths. It was again mild in the early part of the next century, became serious in the middle of that century but subsequently the death rate rapidly fell. Similar trends have been observed with other infectious diseases and there is no reason to assume that they are not still occurring. The vagaries in the mortality rates of infectious disease in the pre-immunisation era should make one careful in attributing changes in the epidemiology of some diseases to the result of specific treatment or immunisation.

Control of Infectious Disease

There is no doubt that the development of immunisation has been one of the most striking features in control of infectious disease in recent years, but immunisation is indicated only when the classic methods of control are impracticable or unsuccessful. For example, if cholera is introduced into the UK or the USA, there is no question of embarking on immunisation, even if there were highly effective vaccine, for cholera is unlikely to spread in these and other industrialized countries because of the high standard of public health practices.

There is no adequate way, other than by immunisation, of controlling diseases which are transmitted by personal contact, such as the common respiratory or enterovirus infections. At the same time, just as surgeons must not forget the importance of asepsis in this antibiotic era, so physicians must not forget the importance of public health methods in the control of common infections. Thus isolation should not be written off as applying only to exotic diseases: contact between old people and children with respiratory diseases should be discouraged, small babies should be protected from being infected by siblings, and patients with influenza should be discouraged from battling to work until all their associates are infected. Good personal hygiene is still important in the prevention of disease. Whether we should use face masks during travel in crowded conditions to prevent the spread of influenza is difficult to decide. Masks have been used during influenza epidemics in the USSR and elsewhere, but there is no evidence of their value and indeed they might make spread of infection easier in some conditions by building up a high concentration of micro-organisms in the masks, which would be readily transmitted during sneezing or coughing or when changing the masks.

Immunisation

Before considering immunisation it must be shown that the disease in question is of sufficient severity, frequency or other importance to justify immunisation against it. Nowadays no one would think of immunising against plague in the UK or USA for there is no risk of infection. There is little good reason for introducing mumps vaccine as a routine procedure, for the disease is usually mild, complications such as pancreatitis and orchitis are rare, and the prognosis of the common complications, namely meningitis and meningoencephalitis, is good. There may be a place for its use in certain circumstances (see Chapter 13) but we must differentiate between selective and routine immunisation. For example, while there is a good vaccine available against anthrax there is no question of making it routinely available; it should be used selectively for those at high risk.

If the infection is readily treatable there is seldom justification for immunisation. I do not think that a very good case can be made for considering immunisation against gonorrhoea, even if there were an effective vaccine. Is immunisation the way to control that disease? Many would find it difficult to explain to ten-year-old children why they were being given a vaccine which implied acceptance, if not approval, of a certain social pathology. However, a gonorrhoea vaccine is something very much of the future, for the natural disease does not produce immunity against reinfection and it will be difficult to improve on the failure of the natural disease to give immunity. The control of gonorrhoea may depend on adequate treatment, education and better contact tracing, and on breaking the chain of infection rather than vaccination.

In addition to having good epidemiological reasons for introducing a vaccine, there must be good evidence that the vaccine is effective and relatively safe. The risk of the disease in question must be greater than the risk of the immunisation procedure. Serious reactions could be acceptable with a vaccine designed to prevent a disease with a high mortality and morbidity, but not with a disease with few serious complications.

It must always be remembered that there is nothing static about immunisation procedures. They depend on the epidemiology of the disease at the time and place in question. What is right in Chicago may not apply to Ibadan.

Immunisation

There are two methods of achieving immunity: by active or passive immunisation.

Active Immunisation

The best type of active immunisation follows a natural infection which may be clinical or subclinical. With many diseases this often gives lifelong protection at little or no cost to the individual or to the community.

Before measles vaccine was introduced, most children suffered a natural attack of the disease and measles was rare in adults because the body retains a 'memory' for many infectious agents which permits it to respond immediately if the agent is met again. The first contact with many infectious agents stimulates the production of antibodies which combine with and neutralize the agent or its toxins and/or sensitizes lymphocytes which are involved in cell-mediated immunity, but it also sets the stage for an immediate response when the infective agent is met again.

In the past, in countries without immunisation programmes and in many developing countries at present, most people have or had natural infections with all three types of poliomyelitis virus. This produced lifelong immunity but exacted a toll of about one paralytic case for every 1,000 or so immunising infections. With smallpox the cost in lives and disfigurements was so great that parents exposed their children to mild cases hoping that they would develop a modified infection and become immune for life. In recent years this practice of actively exposing individuals to infection was in some places quite common, for some parents held German measles 'tea parties' at which susceptible girls were exposed to infectious children in the hope of inducing lifelong immunity against rubella virus.

While most people are naturally actively immunised for life against a host of infectious agents (many of which produce unrecognized infection), there are many infections which do not produce a durable immunity. The lack of durable immunity against some infections is caused by the presence of multiple immunogenic types of the organism. Thus, while there is only one type of measles virus and of mumps virus, there are multiple types of influenza viruses which undergo antigenic changes every few years and thus make prevention exceedingly difficult. The short-lived immunity to some infections probably relates to the fact that they are very superficial and that there is thus little opportunity for the immune mechanisms to be stimulated.

4

Artificial Immunity

Artificial *active* immunisation involves the administration of an antigen which stimulates immunity. These antigens may be in the form of live or inactivated vaccines. Artificial *passive* immunisation is achieved by injecting antibodies in the form of immunoglobulins.

Live Vaccines

Live vaccines consist of either an agent related to the causative micro-organism, as in the case of vaccinia, or of attenuated strains which are similar to the 'wild' strains in that they infect, replicate and immunise but differ in that they do not, or only rarely, cause illness.

Attenuation was first achieved by Pasteur with rabies vaccine, but really came into its own with the development of BCG (which is an attenuated bovine strain of *Mycobacterium tuberculosis*), with the 17D strain of yellow fever virus (for use in areas where the insect vector could not be controlled) and then with poliomyelitis, measles and rubella virus vaccines. After a single dose of these live virus vaccines, immunity like that of a natural infection is produced. (The reason why three doses of oral poliovirus vaccine are given will be discussed later.) The immunity produced by some vaccines is long lasting; with others, like some natural infections, it may be short. Sufficient time has not yet elapsed to predict with certainty the durability of immunity with the live virus vaccines, which are now in common use, such as poliomyelitis, measles and rubella, but with most of them it appears that it will be long lasting. Live vaccines, as the name implies, consist of agents which are living. They infect and replicate and must be treated with respect. They are readily inactivated by light or when held for any length of time at room temperature and should therefore be stored in a refrigerator. They are inactivated by most disinfectants which should therefore not be used to clean the arm when vaccinating.

Inactivated Vaccines

Inactivated vaccines may consist of either suspensions of killed micro-organisms, e.g. whooping cough, typhoid, cholera and inactivated poliomyelitis vaccine, or of products or fractions of the micro-organisms such as the toxoids prepared from the toxins of *Corynebacterium diphtheriae* or *Clostridium tetani*, or of the diffusible fraction of *Bacillus anthracis* or fractions of viruses (split vaccines) which contain that part of the micro-organism which is capable of inducing immunity.

When an active infection occurs or when a live vaccine is being used, the replicating agent provides an antigenic stimulus over many days. To introduce the equivalent antigenic stimulus with one injection of an inactivated vaccine would usually require a great weight of antigen which might produce severe reactions. Thus it has been found convenient to administer such antigens in divided doses. The first dose or doses 'prime' the immune response (primary immunisation) and a population of memory cells are stimulated which provide a better and more rapid response (secondary response) when the antigen is met again. This secondary response occurs when further doses of the vaccine are given as well as when the natural infection is encountered.

While three properly spaced doses of inactivated vaccines are usually used to produce immunity, if the individual has previously been exposed to natural infection with the micro-organism or to immunisation a single injection would usually be sufficient to recall or boost the immunity. The antibody response to inactivated vaccines is usually related to the quantity and potency of the antigen.

Passive Immunity

While active immunisation lasts for a variable period and is often very durable, passive immunity usually lasts for only weeks or months. It is achieved either naturally, by the passage of antibodies over the placenta which is the mechanism by which small babies are protected against infectious disease, or by the injection of immunoglobulins.

It will be recalled that in serum there are five classes of immunoglobulins: IgG is the major one and accounts for about 80 per cent of the total immunoglobulins. It is able to cross the placenta and diffuses readily into tissue spaces. It is responsible for neutralizing toxins (antitoxic antibody) and enhancing phagocytosis (opsonic activity). IgM is a macroglobulin and these are the first antibodies to appear in response to infections; they appear to be particularly important in the agglutination and lysis of bacteria; they do not cross the placenta or diffuse into tissue spaces. They appear to be important in preventing bacteraemias and septicaemias. IgA appears selectively on mucous and epithelial surfaces and is obviously important in protecting the surfaces of the gastrointestinal and respiratory tracts from invasion by micro-organisms. IgE antibodies are involved in allergic conditions and the biological function of IgD is not yet fully established.

These immunoglobulins may be injected as (a) pooled human gamma globulin which will contain antibodies to those diseases which are prevalent in the community; (b) specific gamma globulin prepared (i) from individuals who are either recently convalescent from the disease in question, e.g. varicella, herpes zoster, mumps, etc. or recently revaccinated or boosted, e.g. with vaccinia or with tetanus toxoid or (ii) from animals, usually horses, immunised with, e.g. diphtheria or tetanus toxins or toxoids; (c) convalescent plasma which will contain IgM which is not normally present in the available immunoglobulins because of their method of preparation.

2. Vaccines and Schedules

In this chapter, the types of vaccines which are generally available and suitable schedules for routine immunisation will be outlined.

Live Virus Vaccines (Table 1)

One of the main problems in the production of vaccines is to find a suitable substrate in which to grow the micro-organisms. Thus vaccinia virus for smallpox vaccine is grown on the skin of calves or sheep, the viruses for yellow fever and influenza vaccines in eggs, while those which have been developed since the 1950s are grown in tissue cultures. These consist of layers of cells which have multiplied inside or on the walls of a vessel which contains a nutrient medium. The tissue cultures are inoculated with virus which replicates in the cells and is released into the fluid phase of the culture and this fluid represents the vaccine.

The tissues used for the vaccines must support viral replication to a reasonably high titre to make the production of the vaccine commercially acceptable and they must be free of any contaminating viruses

Table 1. Live vaccines.

Vaccine	Source of substrate for vaccine
Smallpox	Sheep (calves)
Yellow fever	Chick embryo
Influenza	Chick embryo
Poliomyelitis	Monkey kidney cells
Measles	Dog cells or chick embryo
Rubella	Duck, rabbit, dog or human diploid cells
Mumps	Chick embryo
BCG	Bacteriological medium

or other agents. In the early days of poliovirus vaccines, many people were inadvertently given a virus (SV 40) which was present in the monkey kidneys used for the tissue cultures. (SV stands for 'simian virus' and 40 indicates the number of the contaminating viruses of a similar type which is now about 60.)

In the early days of vaccine production in tissue cultures, as many as 60 to 80 per cent of monkeys used were infected with one or other of these 'fellow traveller' viruses. Any tissue culture containing such contaminating viruses must be discarded and the loss of material in the manufacture of some vaccines may be very great. Some viruses, such as SV 40, are oncogenic in certain animals but there is so far no evidence that they have done any harm to individuals given vaccines which had been contaminated with them. The prevalence of these adventitious viruses in monkeys has led to the use of tissue cultures from other mammals such as dogs and rabbits which can be more readily controlled, and to the further use of cultures from duck and chicken embryos. With the increased use of the latter, the number of adventitious viruses found in chickens has continued to grow and methods for their elimination from flocks used for vaccine production has been intensively studied. Until a few years ago most batches of yellow fever virus vaccine contained a 'fellow traveller' chicken virus, but again there is no evidence of its harming those immunised with that vaccine.

The ubiquity of adventitious viruses in various tissues has led some manufacturers to use fully characterized standardized cells, originating from human fetal tissues which have been shown to be free from all detectable extraneous agents. Such cells are diploid and do not exhibit the properties of malignant cells. However, some scientists are still concerned that cell lines derived from human tissues might be carrying 'human cancer viruses' or the agents of 'slow virus infections'. Such agents might be expected to infect man more readily if they came from human tissues than from animal tissues.

The viruses selected for making live vaccines must be sufficiently attenuated so that they will not produce illness in vaccinated individuals, and yet must not be overattenuated so that they will fail to multiply and immunise.

The method of attenuating viruses for vaccines is usually achieved by passage in non-human tissue cultures which tends to select mutants which grow better in the cells of a foreign host and are attenuated for man. The criteria of attenuation of strains suitable for vaccines were established for poliovirus vaccines and similar standards have been followed in the development of the newer vaccines.

Immunisation

The agents of live vaccines must be genetically stable. If they are excreted and transmitted to contacts they must remain attenuated. Tests of attenuation and safety are carried out in animals, but the final evaluation of safety and effectiveness of all human vaccines must be in man.

The strain of the only live bacterial vaccine in common use, namely BCG, was similarly attenuated by prolonged passage in suitable bacterial cultures.

Inactivated Virus Vaccines

As far as inactivated virus vaccines are concerned, similar care has to be taken of the cultures used for growing the viruses, but they need not be attenuated because they will be inactivated by treating the culture fluids with formalin or other chemicals, or by splitting the antigenic component from the virus particle. As a result of inactivation processes, the chance of having a live extraneous agent in activated vaccines is obviously less than in live vaccines.

Table 2. Advantages and disadvantages of live and inactivated vaccines[1].

Advantages	Disadvantages
Live vaccines:	
Single dose given by natural route. Invokes full range of immunological responses, local IgA as well as systemic antibody production leading to possibility of local eradication of wild-type viruses.	Reversion to virulence dangerous if there is natural spread to contacts. Contaminating viruses, which may include 'human cancer viruses'. Viral interference may prevent infection by vaccine. Inactivation in tropical climates.
Inactivated vaccines:	
Potential of single dose of vaccines. Stability.	Multiple doses and boosters needed: given by injection. High concentration of antigens needed: production difficulties.

[1] Adapted from Fenner et al. (1974), *The Biology of Animal Viruses*, 2nd ed., Academic Press, New York, London.

Inactivated bacterial vaccines are prepared by inactivating suspensions of the bacteria, by treating their toxins with formalin to form toxoids, or by preparing extracts of the bacteria.

Each vaccine, live or inactivated, has had its problems. These will be discussed under the individual vaccines, but in general, the problems encountered with live vaccines are mainly concerned with safety while those of inactivated vaccines relate mainly to efficacy. Both types of vaccines may sometimes present problems of untoward reactions.

The advantages and disadvantages of live and inactivated vaccines are shown in Table 2. There are qualifications which could be added, but the points form a useful basis for the subsequent discussions of individual vaccines.

Schedules of Routine Immunisation

Various schedules of immunisation have been proposed, but only those recommended in the UK and in the USA will be discussed here. Schedules involving quadruple vaccine, as used in Canada, are outlined in Chapter 7 and those suitable for developing countries in Chapter 15.

United Kingdom

The schedule for routine immunisation outlined in Table 3 is a general guide recommended by the Department of Health and Social Security in England. This schedule may not meet every case, but there are considerable advantages in having uniformity of procedure so that when children move from one place to another and change their doctors they will not be involved in a different course of immunisation.

Since it is still necessary to immunise against diphtheria, whooping cough and poliomyelitis, it is desirable to provide the highest protection to the preschool child, in whom there is the highest risk of contracting or spreading these diseases. Although tetanus is rare in the UK, it is commonest in children, and it is convenient to include that vaccine with those of diphtheria and pertussis.

The starting time for the schedule outlined in Table 3 is fairly flexible but recently in the hope of improving the efficacy of immunisation against whooping cough (see Chapter 5), the majority of the Joint Committee on Vaccination and Immunisation of the DHSS have recommended that routine immunisation with dip/tet/pert should commence at three months. Personally I think that there are good reasons for delaying immunisation against diphtheria, tetanus, pertussis

Table 3. Recommended schedule for active routine immunisation of normal individuals in the United Kingdom[1].

Age	Vaccine	Interval	Notes
During the first year of life	Dip/tet/pert and oral polio vaccine (first dose)		The earliest age at which the first dose should be given is three months, but a better general immunological response can be expected if the first dose is delayed to six months of age
	Dip/tet/pert and oral polio vaccine (second dose)	Preferably after an interval of six to eight weeks	
	Dip/tet/pert and oral polio vaccine (third dose)	Preferably after an interval of four to six months	
During the second year of life	Measles vaccine	After an interval of not less than three weeks	Although measles vaccination can be given in the second year of life, delay until three years of age or more will reduce the risk of occasional severe reactions to the vaccine which occur mainly in children under the age of three years
At five years of age or school entry	Dip/tet and oral polio vaccine or dip/tet/polio vaccine		
Between 10 and 13 years of age	BCG vaccine		These may be given, if desired, at three years of age to children entering nursery schools, attending day nurseries or living in children's homes
All girls aged 11 to 13 years	Rubella vaccine	There should be an interval of not less than three weeks between BCG and rubella vaccination	All girls of this age should be offered rubella vaccine whether or not there is a past history of an attack of rubella
At 15 to 19 years of age or on leaving school	Polio vaccine (oral or inactivated) and tetanus toxoid		

[1] Data from Immunisation Against Infectious Diseases (1972), DHSS, London.

and poliomyelitis until the second half of the first year of life in children in industrialised countries.

In the first place infection with these diseases is rare in babies under six months of age in developed countries. (Although whooping cough deaths tend to be concentrated in small babies, as will be discussed in Chapter 5, many people consider that the greatest protection of them will be achieved by immunising the older siblings and thus reducing the likelihood of transmitting the bacteria to babies.)

Second, the presence of maternally transmitted antibody masks the antigenic effect of certain vaccines. Thus when mothers have acquired antibody (naturally or by active immunisation), it is usually transmitted to the baby. This inhibits the antigenic effect of vaccines given in the early months of life. It is sometimes possible to overcome this effect by giving larger doses of the vaccines, but this is unacceptable because of the reactions which might occur. Furthermore, large doses of concentrated vaccines would be too costly for routine use. Most maternal antibodies gradually disappear during the first six months of the baby's life. However, measles antibody can still have an inhibiting effect up to 12 months of age—one reason why measles vaccine is not recommended until the second year of life.

Third, small babies are less immunologically mature than older ones. Although babies can respond to antigenic stimuli from a very early age, the immunity mechanism, particularly that of cell mediated immunity, is incompletely developed in the newborn.

Finally reactions to some vaccines are more frequent in small babies than in older ones and are also less often recognized. In one study of dip/tet/pert vaccine conducted in the early 1960s, there were 23 major reactions (screaming, collapse, etc.), following 495 inoculations in babies of less than six months, and only one in 471 inoculations in older babies. Modern pertussis vaccines are much less reactogenic.

Reactions to vaccines are unacceptable, not only because of the possible damage to the baby, but because the greater the number or severity of reactions, the larger will be the number of defaulters from completing the course.

Some say that if immunisation is delayed, the 'captive baby' will be lost. This really applies only to babies attending maternal and child welfare clinics. It is possible that some clinics are too rigidly organized, or have computer programmes which they do not care to change. With the DHSS schedule using the triple antigen, the only good reason for starting immunisation much before six months would appear to me to be an administrative one.

Immunisation

Many suggest that immunisation should be the responsibility of the general practitioner who knows the baby and any contraindications to immunisation which may exist in a particular child.

Spacing of Doses

The recommended interval between the first and second dose of dip/tet/pert and poliovirus vaccine is six to eight weeks (Table 3). This is advantageous for oral polio vaccines (q.v.) as well as for dip/tet/pert and it is administratively convenient to give them at the same time. If the first and second doses of tetanus and diphtheria toxoids are closely spaced, then the second dose makes very little contribution to the ultimate antibody response. It appears that durable immunity will be obtained if the third dose is given about six months after the second. An easy schedule for doctors and mothers to remember is to start at six months, second dose six weeks later, third dose six months later. Following this schedule, no further immunisation against diphtheria, tetanus, whooping cough or polio is required until school entry. At that time a booster of dip/tet and poliovirus vaccines, but not pertussis vaccine, should be given.

If immunisation with dip/tet/pert is started before three months and if the intervals between the three injections are about one month, it may be necessary to give a booster of dip/tet/pert at 16 to 18 months. Those who support this latter programme usually fail to give the 16 to 18 months booster dose of vaccine. The three-month starting date is also less satisfactory for immunisation against poliomyelitis than commencing at about six months.

Other Vaccines

The proposed times of immunising against measles, rubella and BCG are shown in Table 3. An interval of about three weeks should be allowed between giving two live vaccines (e.g. polio, measles, smallpox and yellow fever). The reason for this is concerned with sorting out problems of reactions in some individuals rather than of any interference of the vaccine viruses.

Interrupted Programme

If the immunisation programme has been started at six months and the first two doses have been given but the third dose has not been given at about six months later, then it is probable that if the third dose is given up to 12 months later, it will be effective in most cases. If only the first dose has been given at about six months, then two doses at about six months' interval should be adequate to complete the course.

United States of America

The schedule which is recommended for healthy infants and children in the USA by the American Academy of Pediatrics is outlined in Table 4. Like the one recommended in the UK this is suggested as a guide which may require modification for certain individual or group requirements.

The Public Health Service Advisory Committee on Immunisation Practices (US Department of Health, Education and Welfare) recommends that immunisation with dip/tet/pert should begin at two to three months of age or at the six-week check-up, and that three doses should be given at four to eight-week intervals, and a fourth dose approximately one year after the third. The primary course recommended for polio immunisation is one of three doses, the first two doses preferably eight weeks apart, and the third dose eight to 12 months later. (The first dose is commonly given at the same time as the first dose of dip/tet/pert.) It will be noted that the age for beginning immunisation is somewhat earlier than in the UK.

Hazards of Immunisation

Every vaccine carries certain hazards and can produce untoward reactions in some people. The importance of these reactions has to be weighed against the consequences of a natural infection. If the risk of being seriously incapacitated by a disease is high, severe reactions to the vaccine concerned are more acceptable than if the disease is mild and of little consequence. It is difficult to arrive at precise estimates of the risks associated with some immunisation procedures but, in general, there are more vaccine complications than is generally appreciated.

Doctors are reluctant to consider an illness following immunisation as being caused by something which they have recommended and have often persuaded the mother to accept for her baby. Local reactions will be obvious, but a complication of a severe nature occurring within 6 to 12 hours or 8 to 10 days after vaccination may not be considered as being vaccine associated. Where the known incidence of some of the reactions which follow immunisations may be of the order of 1:100,000, the physician may not have previously seen such a complication and may not associate it with immunisation.

Table 4. Recommended schedule for active routine immunisation of normal individuals in the USA[1].

Age	Vaccine	Notes
2 months	Dip/tet/pert and oral polio vaccine	Suitable for breast-fed as well as bottle-fed babies
4 months	Dip/tet/pert and oral polio vaccine	
6 months	Dip/tet/pert and oral polio vaccine	
1 year	Measles, rubella, mumps, tuberculin test	May be given at 1 year as combined measles – rubella or measles – mumps – rubella vaccines
Measles vaccine may be given at 6 months in places where measles frequent in first year of life. In such circumstances a repeat dose should be given at 1 year.
Frequency of repeated tuberculin tests depends on risk of exposure and prevalence of tuberculosis. Initial test should be at time of, or preceding, measles immunisation.
$1\frac{1}{2}$ years	Dip/tet/pert and oral polio vaccine	
4 to 6 years	Dip/tet/pert and oral polio vaccine	
14 to 16 years	Tet	And every 10 years thereafter

[1] Data from *Report of the Committee on Infectious Diseases* (1974), 17th edition, American Academy of Pediatrics, Evanston, Illinois.

It is important that practitioners should be aware of the known hazards which occur with the various vaccines. All reactions which follow the administration of any vaccines (whether considered to be caused by the vaccine or not) should be immediately reported. In the UK this notification should be made to the Committee on Safety of Medicines, and preferably also to the local district or community physician until a more suitable mechanism for making these reports is organized. In the USA reactions should be reported to the Center for

Disease Control (CDC), US Public Health Service, Department of Health, Education and Welfare, Atlanta, Georgia 30333. Although CDC is principally a resource for local and State Departments it also offers direct and indirect services to practising physicians and hospitals in the USA.

Contraindications

Special contraindications to individual vaccines will be discussed separately, but the following contraindications apply to all vaccines used for elective immunisation.

Vaccines should not be given to babies or children who are not in good health. The proposed schedules are sufficiently flexible to allow postponement of any of the doses. If a child has a severe reaction following a dose of vaccine, then the risk of a similar or more severe reaction following a subsequent dose must be considered. Some irritability and fever follows some immunisations. This would not normally be considered a contraindication but the onset of convulsions or other serious reactions should be a contraindication to further immunisation.

Live virus vaccines should not be given to individuals with immunological deficiencies or those receiving steroid therapy, immunosuppressive drugs or radiotherapy. They should not be given to those suffering from malignant conditions, e.g. lymphoma, leukaemia, Hodgkin's disease or other tumours of the reticuloendothelial system. Live vaccines should not be given routinely to pregnant women, because of possible harm to the fetus. Their administration should be deferred until about three months after passive immunisation.

Surveillance

We must be prepared to carry out continuous surveillance of immunisation procedures. The usefulness of a vaccine may decrease with time, because of changes in the epidemiological pattern of the disease or in the formulation of the vaccine. The effectiveness of vaccine surveillance depends on the accuracy of reporting of the diseases and of vaccine complications and on serological surveys or other field trials of the vaccines in use.

3. Diphtheria

Active immunisation against diphtheria, which will be discussed in this chapter, is carried out with diphtheria toxoid. This consists of the toxin of *Corynebacterium diphtheriae*, which has been rendered non-toxigenic but has retained its antigenicity. This toxoid is usually given routinely as a triple vaccine which contains about 25Lf[1] diphtheria toxoid, 5Lf tetanus toxoid and not more than 20×10^9 killed *Bordetella pertussis* with or without a mineral carrier. Passive immunisation is considered in Chapter 14.

Historical

In the 18th and 19th centuries deaths from scarlet fever were in excess of those of diphtheria, but by the late 1800s diphtheria was the most important cause of death in children (Figure 1). From 1870 to 1900 there was little change in the mortality, but since then there has been a continuous and unbroken decline. The reason for the drop in diphtheria mortality in the 1900s was presumably the result of the introduction of antisera towards the end of the last century.

At the beginning of the century Behring and his colleagues in Germany showed that diphtheria was caused by a toxin formed by *Corynebacterium diphtheriae* rather than by invasion of the tissues and that *C. diphtheriae* was capable of stimulating the production of a specific neutralizing antitoxin in the blood and tissue fluids on which immunity to the disease was largely dependent. Not only did these

---

[1] The Lf dose of toxin is determined by titration against the standard international antitoxin. L means limit and f means flocculation. The Lf unit of toxin is the amount of toxin which gives the most rapid flocculation with one unit of antitoxin.

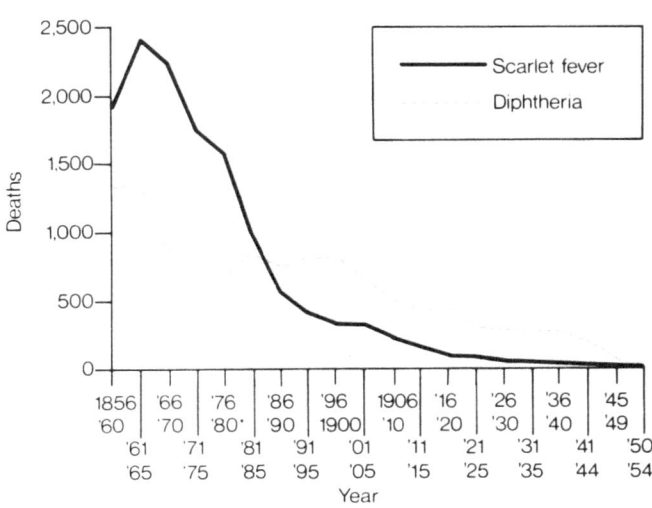

Figure 1. *Deaths from scarlet fever and diphtheria per million under 15 years of age: 1856–1954.*

observations lead to the development of antisera for treatment, which influenced the case fatality rate, but also to the development of toxoid vaccines. The use of toxoid vaccines were pioneered in the USA by W. H. Park and led to a drop from 100,000 cases each year with 15,000 deaths before 1925 to 307 notified cases in 1975 with only 5 deaths.

It is surprising that the acceptance of this highly effective immunisation procedure against diphtheria was so long delayed in Britain. The Ministry of Health had been advocating active immunisation with toxoid since the early 1920s, but for the next 20 years the medical profession showed little enthusiasm for using the vaccine against a disease which in England and Wales was killing 2,000 to 3,000 children annually. It can only be assumed that the failure of government propaganda to encourage immunisation was due to a lack of confidence in the vaccine because there had been a few mishaps associated with its use in the USA and in some countries in Europe. Today it seems remarkable that the profession did not weigh these few mishaps against the tens of thousands of cases which were occurring every year.

In 1941 extensive programmes of immunisation were begun in the UK. There followed a dramatic fall in the notifications and in the number of deaths from diphtheria (Figure 2). The disease has now virtually disappeared from the UK and other countries with active

Immunisation

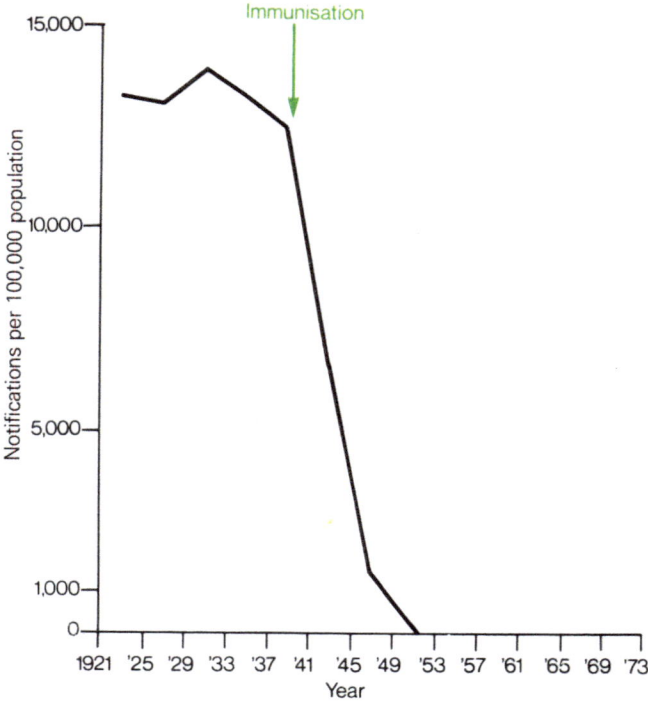

Figure 2. *Notifications of diphtheria in England and Wales per 100,000 population.*

immunisation programmes using potent diphtheria toxoids. In 1953 there were only 23 deaths in England and Wales (1 in 1,000,000 population). Table 5 shows the number of deaths in recent years.

Herd Immunity

In the past, many adults were immune as a result of childhood infections. Diphtheria tended to disappear from communities where about 75 per cent of the preschool and school children had been immunised. This 75 per cent figure has often been used as a goal for all immunisations and its significance is not always understood. When diphtheria was prevalent in the UK its 'reproduction rate' was about four, i.e. each infected person could in theory give rise to an average of four cases. This rate depends on many factors, but the disease must die out when the reproduction rate becomes less than one. This happened in the late

20

1940s in the UK when about 75 per cent of the susceptible population were immunised. This 75 per cent rate applies to diphtheria only in the epidemiological and social background of the 1940s.

There is nothing magical in trying to achieve a 75 per cent immunisation rate in the prevention of other diseases. Poliomyelitis and measles have much higher reproduction rates and it is obvious that higher immunisation rates will be required for their disappearance. On the other hand smallpox has disappeared from communities where only 50 to 60 per cent of the population has been vaccinated.

Present Position

The better implementation of immunisation programmes has now eliminated the occasional outbreaks which centred around schools in the early 1960s in the UK. Outbreaks which have occurred in the past ten or so years have been located in hospitals for the mentally handicapped or have been introduced by immigrants.

In 1953 there were only 23 deaths from diphtheria in England and Wales (0.5 per 1,000,000 population). Table 5 shows the number of deaths in recent years. In the USA there were 137 deaths from 1966 to 1970 and only 43 between 1971 and 1975: as indicated, the number of reported cases remains at between 150 and 800, all in localized outbreaks in many parts of the USA. Many of these cases have been severe.

Now that there is little clinical diphtheria in the UK, diphtheria bacilli are rarely isolated by laboratories, and those which are recovered are usually non-toxigenic. It will be remembered that there are three types of *Corynebacteria diphtheriae*: *gravis* and *intermedius*, which are usually associated with a case fatality rate of about eight per cent, and *mitis* with a rate of three per cent. In addition to these rare isolations of non-toxigenic strains of *Corynebacteria*, strains of other species, *C. ulcerans* and *C. haemolyticum*, have recently been recovered from patients with membranous tonsillitis accompanied by an irritant rash.

Many doctors have never seen a case of diphtheria and if they do, it may well be atypical (e.g. a *gravis* infection in an immunised person may look more like tonsillitis than diphtheria). A history of immunisation

Table 5. Number of deaths caused by diphtheria (England and Wales).

1954–58	1959–63	1964–68	1969–73
39	17	6	4

21

must not lead the physician to rule out a diagnosis of diphtheria.

Once diphtheria has ceased to be endemic in any country, consideration should be given to abandoning routine immunisation as has been done in the case of smallpox vaccine in the UK and USA.

Although there are now high rates of immunisation of children in the UK the adult population is only about 20 to 50 per cent immune as measured by the Schick test[1]. There is some evidence to suggest that this rate is falling, mainly because there are no pathogenic strains of *C. diphtheriae* circulating in the community which could boost the immunity. With this low rate of immunity in adults and no bacilli to boost artificial immunity, why does diphtheria not re-emerge when it is imported?

Diphtheria is essentially a carrier-borne disease. Importations can occur silently and a focus of infection could develop before the disease was recognized clinically. Diphtheria may not have re-emerged in developed countries because the facility for spread of diphtheria among adults is much less than among children. Children are quantitatively better transmitters of bacteria and viruses than adults and also the method of spread of diphtheria may be less likely to occur among adults than children. If this is so, the reproduction rate in adults is presumably less than in children, perhaps only one or two. Therefore, nowadays quite a low rate of immunity in adults may be sufficient to prevent the spread of diphtheria if high rates of immunisation are maintained in children.

The immune rate in adults may be much higher than appears from

---

[1] Schick test: If diphtheria toxin is injected intradermally (i.d.) into a susceptible (non-immune) person it produces local damage. If the individual is immune the toxin is neutralized and produces no reaction. In the Schick test 0.2 ml of diphtheria toxoid is injected (i.d.) into the left forearm and as a control heated toxin is injected into the right forearm.

1. There may be no reaction in either arm—a negative result which means that the patient had sufficient circulating antitoxin to neutralize the injected toxin and is immune.

2. There may be a reaction in the left arm which appears one to two days after the injection and consists mainly of an area of erythema at the injection site which reaches its maximum diameter of 2 to 5 cm in about four or five days, may persist for a couple of weeks and eventually becomes brown in colour. This staining may persist for several weeks. This is a positive reaction and the patient is susceptible and should be immunised if considered necessary. A slightly more complicated result may be obtained: diphtheria toxoid is prepared from cultures of *C. diphtheriae* and the test material may contain bacterial products (other than toxin) to which the patient may be hypersensitive. This hypersensitivity reaction appears within about 12 hours (earlier than the positive reaction and fades within three to

Schick testing, for although individuals are Schick negative when the blood contains less than 0.01 units antitoxin per millilitre, those with lower levels may nevertheless be immune. Since diphtheria toxoid rarely causes serious harm (although it can occasionally give an unpleasant reaction) and since immunisation can be carried out with little trouble with the combined vaccine, it would seem reasonable to continue immunising. Although the disease has virtually disappeared in countries like the UK, it is still present in many other parts of the world. In these areas, active programmes of immunisation are most essential.

Routine Immunisation

In addition to routine infant immunisation with triple antigen a reinforcing dose of dip/tet toxoid should be given at school entry (see Schedules, Chapter 2).

High Risk Groups

In the past the disease was most serious in young children. Today those at high risk are not children but nursing staff and patients in homes for the mentally handicapped. Any patient admitted to such an institute and all nursing and other staff working in these homes should receive booster injections or a complete course of immunisation if they have not previously received one. Reinforcing doses of toxoids are recommended for those working in countries where there is still a high inci-

---

four days). It is produced equally well by the test, and by the control material, for the products producing this reaction are heat stable. This type of reaction is called a pseudoreaction.

3. If there are identical pseudoreactions in both arms it means that the patient is reacting to the products of C. diphtheriae and has had a subclinical or a clinical infection in the past and is immune. If he had not been sensitive to the products of the Corynebacteria he would have shown a negative reaction. Such a patient should not be immunised and might react violently if he were given toxoid.

4. Occasionally there may be a combined reaction in which the hypersensitivity reaction is superimposed on a positive reaction, so that the reactions in both arms start in about 24 hours and while the left arm proceeds to a positive reaction the right arm fades as in a pseudoreaction. It would appear that such a patient is positive, that is, he has no circulating antitoxin but is susceptible to the products of C. diphtheriae. In point of fact, sensitive in vitro tests show that the sera from such patients do contain antitoxin but at a level below that detected by the i.d. test; the fact that they show the pseudoreactions indicates previous infection with C. diphtheriae and that they will probably react violently to toxoid and should therefore not be immunised.

dence of the disease, e.g. in countries of the Indian subcontinent such as Nepal.

Vaccines Used

The instructions of the manufacturer with regard to doses should be carefully followed.

Diphtheria Toxoid

For children under 10 years of age purified diphtheria toxoids are poor antigens. For the basic course of immunisation they require the adjuvant effect of combination with aluminium phosphate or aluminium hydroxide (adsorbed toxoids) or to be combined with *B. pertussis* as in the triple vaccine.

Where previous immunisation with dip/tet/pert vaccine has produced a reaction, adsorbed toxoid in combination with tetanus toxoid is suitable for completing the course of immunisation and also for the courses of immunisation by those who do not subscribe to the use of vaccines containing a pertussis component (q.v.).

For reinforcement of immunity at school entry, either the adsorbed vaccine or a mixture of dip/tet without a mineral carrier may be used. This latter vaccine is not suitable for the primary course.

If primary immunisation or if a reinforcing dose is to be given to a child over 10 years of age or to an adult, a preliminary Schick test is indicated to avoid giving the vaccine to those who are immune (i.e. those showing a negative or pseudocombined reaction). Because 'wild' strains are rare today, negative or pseudoreactions are much less frequently found in non-immunised children than in the past. Toxoid containing an aluminium adjuvant is again preferable for these immunisations.

Site of Injections

The triple vaccine or any of its components should be inoculated intramuscularly by a deep subcutaneous injection into the middle third of the deltoid or triceps (except when a booster dose is given intradermally). Inoculations into the upper and outer quadrant of the buttock or vastus lateralis are recommended by some, but my impression is that such inoculations are associated with more discomfort and more reactions in children. The swabbing of a clean baby's arm before injection is purely ritualistic! (If spirit is used it often causes stinging if the spirit is not allowed to dry.)

The vaccine for reinforcing immunity to diphtheria and tetanus at school entry may be given intradermally (i.d.), but any vaccine preparation given i.d. must not contain a mineral carrier.

Reactions

General reactions after immunisation of children with diphtheria toxoid or dip/tet toxoids are usually mild. Sometimes there is slight pyrexia and malaise. There may be some local swelling at the site of inoculation and erythema may persist for a few days. With all adsorbed vaccines, a hard nodule may persist at the site of inoculation for at least a week or two (the more obvious are usually associated with more superficial injections). Reactions are usually more severe in adults.

Occasionally an allergic reaction may follow the injection of diphtheria toxoid manifested by pallor and dyspnoea. This requires the immediate subcutaneous injection of 0.5 ml of 1:1,000 adrenaline solution. Although most doctors may never see such an allergic reaction, all physicians engaged in immunisation should have adrenaline at hand so that an immediate injection may be given if required.

Since some adults and adolescents may react violently to diphtheria toxoid it is advisable, as already indicated, to perform a Schick test before giving booster doses and to vaccinate only the reactors.

Storage

The box of vaccine should be placed in a cool part of a refrigerator (2 to 10° C) on receipt and always stored there after use. Although some vaccines are supplied in rubber capped bottles, individual ampoules are preferable for all immunisations.

Contraindications

As already mentioned any child who is unwell, who has a history of allergy or convulsions, should not be immunised.

4. Tetanus

Immunisation against tetanus can have no influence on the natural history of the disease, for *Clostridium tetani* is found in the faeces of horses, cows, sheep and other animals, including man. It is particularly prevalent in soil in agricultural areas but the spores of tetanus bacilli can occur anywhere. These spores are highly resistant and can contaminate almost any substance including many items used in medicine. Like *Corynebacterium diphtheriae, Cl. tetani* makes an exotoxin which produces the disease. Prevention of the disease is achieved by active immunisation with toxoid or passive immunisation with antitetanus immunoglobulins. A natural attack of tetanus does not produce immunity.

While classical tetanus is associated with dirty lacerated or punctured wounds, 40 or 50 per cent of cases of tetanus result from wounds which are so trivial that medical attention has not been sought. In as many as one-third of the cases, there has been no detectable wound. It is obvious that if tetanus is to be prevented, it is no use putting reliance on prophylaxis at the time of injury.

Incidence

Tetanus is relatively uncommon in most industrialized countries. The mortality from tetanus depends on the speed and efficacy of treatment which should be carried out in special centres which have the necessary equipment and expertise. It is an important cause of death in rural tropical areas in South America, Africa and Asia.

In many countries deaths are reported from 'tetanus' or from 'injury complicated by tetanus'. Table 6 shows reported cases in England and Wales from 1955 to 1970. The actual figures may be higher because a death in which an injury has been complicated by tetanus may be notified as simply being caused by an accident. With modern methods, the case fatality rate is probably 20 per cent, so that today there may be about 100 cases of tetanus each year in England and Wales. Throughout the world, there are probably 100,000 deaths from tetanus each year; 30 per cent of these are in the newborn which have resulted from contamination of the umbilical stump. These are preventable by immunising mothers. In developed countries tetanus is uncommonly diagnosed in infants and small children and the highest incidence appears to be among children of school age. However, a growing proportion of cases seem to be occurring among older people, e.g. gardeners who have had a trivial injury. Although the disease cannot be regarded as a major public health problem in developed countries, there should be even fewer cases with proper use of the preventive and prophylactic techniques available.

Table 6. Reported cases of tetanus in England and Wales: 1955 to 1970.

	1955	1960	1965	1970
Tetanus	33	18	21	9
Complicated by tetanus	15	14	12	15
All deaths	48	32	33	24

Immunisation

Routine infant immunisation against tetanus is purely for the protection of the individual and has no community value, because it will not eliminate the organism.

Recent active immunisation is effective in the prevention of the disease. However, if a person who has been actively immunised is exposed to the danger of tetanus, a reinforcing dose of toxoid at the time of injury will usually produce a rapid boost of circulating antitoxin which will afford protection. The objective of routine immunisation is to provide a basic immunity in the entire population which can be boosted at intervals throughout life and at the time of an injury suspected of being contaminated with *Cl. tetani*.

Individuals who have not been immunised as babies should be immunised as school leavers or students or on entering employment. Those at high risk such as manual labourers, road workers, mechanics, farm workers, etc. should be given a basic course of immunisation and adequate boosters.

Immunisation

Routine Infant Immunisation

Tetanus toxoid is more effective when adsorbed on aluminium hydroxide. It may be given with diphtheria toxoid and *Bordetella pertussis* (the triple vaccine) or with diphtheria toxoid only. In general, the adsorbed toxoid produces a more durable immune response than simple fluid toxoid. The interval between doses for the basic course of immunisation of infants has been discussed in Chapter 2.

Reactions to the tetanus component of the combined antigen are rare in infants and children and the reactions to dip/tet and dip/tet/pert are discussed in Chapters 3 and 5.

Reinforcement of Immunity

A reinforcing dose of dip/tet vaccine should be given at school entry. Again a vaccine with a mineral carrier is preferred.

A dose of tetanus toxoid (adsorbed) is recommended on leaving school and, as always, the dose of vaccine advised by the manufacturer should be followed. Reactions are rare but there may be some local swelling and pain at the site of inoculation. Individuals who have reacted to previous reinforcing doses may be given 0.1 ml of non-adsorbed simple toxoid intradermally.

Immunisation of Adults

The adsorbed toxoid is again preferred and three doses of vaccine should be given with an interval of not less than six weeks between the first and second dose and of about six to 12 months between the second and third doses. Persons who react to the first dose may be given a half dose of simple non-adsorbed fluid toxoid for the second and third doses. Alternatively, the course may be completed with simple fluid toxoid in 0.1 ml doses intradermally.

The intradermal route seems to have about a three to five times adjuvant effect so that a dose of 0.1 ml i.d. will have about the same antigenic effect as 0.5 ml given by the subcutaneous route. *The adsorbed vaccine must not be given i.d.* While simple toxoid may be used for booster doses, all evidence suggests that the adsorbed toxoid produces a more durable immunity and should always be used for primary immunisation. It is simpler to have only one preparation at hand and the adsorbed toxoid is the one of choice—three doses of fluid toxoid give a far less durable response than is obtained with two doses of the same toxoid adsorbed on aluminium phosphate.

Duration of Immunity and Boosters

The duration of immunity depends on the potency of the toxoid used and on the careful spacing of the primary doses and boosters. Following the schedules described, in the normal course of events boosters should not be required at intervals of less than ten years. Indeed, it may well be that an individual who has been immunised with potent vaccine as a baby and has had a reinforcing dose at school entry and school leaving will be immune for life.

This may not apply universally. In developing countries, for example, perhaps as a result of malnutrition, babies may be less capable of responding to certain antigens and immunity may fall away faster in such individuals than in babies and children in highly developed areas (see Chapter 15).

Reactions

Reactions to immunisation increase with age and with the frequency of reinforcing doses in those at high risk. Fluid toxoid is less reactogenic than adsorbed toxoid but it is also less antigenic. The incidence of reactions in adults is probably in the region of one per cent. There may be local swelling, pain and redness within a few hours of immunisation which usually passes off in three or four days, but sometimes what appears to be an Arthus type of reaction[1] develops about 10 days after inoculation with considerable local tenderness and malaise. Rarely there may be frank 'serum sickness' with onset about 10 days after inoculation. However, the commonest type of general reaction is urticaria with or without angioneurotic oedema. Individuals who develop reactions and require reinforcing doses should be given simple fluid toxoid intradermally.

Prophylaxis After Injury

In conclusion one must mention immunisation in the prevention of tetanus after a potentially contaminated wound. In the few cases where serum therapy is indicated it is best to use specific human antitetanus

---

[1] Arthus-type reaction. When there is an excess of antigen the complexes formed by antigen and antibody may be toxic to the tissues, for example, in serum sickness where large amounts of foreign serum proteins (antigen) are circulating and antibody is beginning to be produced but is immediately combined with the antigen as it enters the circulation; or when antibody is present in the blood and when high concentrations of antigen are injected into the tissue as in repeated injections of tetanus toxoids. In this type 3 reaction, the antigen–antibody complexes cause damage to the intima of small blood vessels.

immunoglobulin. More and more doctors now accept the recommendation that the prophylaxis of tetanus involves the use of tetanus toxoid. Because of the medicolegal position, antitetanus serum (ATS) continued to be used for many years after it was realized that it was harmful, and indeed the number of deaths from ATS therapy in the UK (perhaps about 1:200,000) exceeded those from tetanus.

A simple guide to active and passive tetanus immunisation at the time of wound cleansing and debridement, as recommended by the Advisory Committee on Immunisation Practices of the US Public Health Service, is outlined in Table 7. This schedule presumes a reliable knowledge of the patient's history.

Table 7. Guide to tetanus prophylaxis in wound management[1].

History of tetanus immunisation	Clean minor wounds		All other wounds	
	Tet/toxoid	Specific tet immuno-globulin (human)	toxoid	tet immuno-globulin (human)
Dose				
Uncertain	Yes	No	Yes	Yes
0–1	Yes	No	Yes	Yes
2	Yes	No	Yes	No[2]
3 or more	No[3]	No	No[4]	No

[1] Data from US Public Health Service Advisory Committee on Immunisation Practices (1977), MMWR, **26**, 49.
[2] Unless wound more than 24 hours old.
[3] Unless more than 10 years since last dose.
[4] Unless more than 5 years since last dose.

It should be emphasized that all wounds are susceptible to tetanus and that they must be thoroughly cleansed of devitalized tissue and foreign material. For individuals who have had a complete course of immunisation (four doses of toxoid), it is unnecessary to give booster injections more than once every five years in wound management. If needed, 0.5 ml tetanus toxoid (adsorbed) should be given. In a first course of immunisation the second dose of tetanus toxoid should be given about six weeks later and a third in six to twelve months' time. If the wound is penetrating, extensive and very dirty and cannot be adequately cleansed, or was sustained more than six hours previously, a dose of specific human antitetanus immunoglobulin should be given into the other arm. In wounds which cannot have complete debridement and where there are likely to be problems of healing, chemotherapy may also be used.

Records

The most reliable and effective method of protecting the population against tetanus is to ensure that all are immunised. It would seem sensible that actively immunised adolescents and adults should carry a card recording their vaccination status.

Occasional failures have been recorded following primary immunisation, but in these it is often difficult to assess the efficacy of the primary course. It seems clear, however, that a recommended course will, with rare exceptions, supply the necessary basic immunity so that boosters given at the time of injury will provide complete protection.

5. Whooping Cough

Without laboratory confirmation, the certain diagnosis of whooping cough may be difficult, and the ability of laboratories to isolate *Bordetella pertussis* from what appear to be typical cases shows enormous variation.

Diagnosis

Some of the failures of bacteriology laboratories to isolate *B. pertussis* may stem from the provision of unsatisfactory specimens. Probably the best method of specimen collection is to hold a bacteriological plate containing the special Bordet–Gengou medium in front of the mouth of a coughing child. These 'cough plates' must be taken to the laboratory as soon as possible. Alternatively a pernasal swab of the nasopharynx should be taken by passing the swab (made with fine flexible fibre) along the floor of one nostril to the nasopharynx. A West's swab may also be used. The cotton wool of this swab is attached to a piece of fibre housed inside a piece of curved plastic tubing which is open at both ends. The curved end is passed up behind the soft palate and the swab is pushed up into the nasopharynx. It is then withdrawn into the plastic tube which is removed and taken immediately to the laboratory. I have never found this easy to manipulate in infants. Higher recovery rates appear to be obtained using Augur suction to obtain secretions.

While failure to isolate *B. pertussis* may be a technical one, there are some viruses, e.g. adenoviruses, parainfluenza viruses and respiratory syncytial virus (RSV), which may give rise to an infection which in some respects may resemble that caused by *B. pertussis*. In some children other viruses may be present with *B. pertussis* and it is possible that the severity of infection with *B. pertussis* may be potentiated by the secondary virus infection or vice versa. Since it is realized that some reappraisal of the aetiology of paroxysmal coughs in small children is required, physicians should make more use of the bacteriological and virological laboratory facilities available for confirmation of their diagnoses. They will thus become more skilled in the exact aetiological diagnosis of the conditions. It is always best to discuss the collection of specimens with the bacteriologist.

The diagnosis of mild infections may be difficult. If the characteristic whoop has not been heard the clinical diagnosis may sometimes rest on a persistent cough which often occurs at night and is sometimes associated with vomiting. The common complications are bronchopneumonia and collapse of the lung and very rarely cerebral anoxia with potential brain damage.

Bronchiectasis as a complication appears to be a thing of the past in industrialized countries and presumably this is due to better therapy of secondary bronchopneumonia. However, severe infections *can* occur, particularly in the very young. For some years the case fatality rate in the UK has been about 1 in 1,000 notified cases (Figure 3). A similar fatality rate (less than 0.5 per cent) applies in the USA.

In the UK and USA whooping cough outbreaks usually last for about two years at intervals of roughly three or four years, but sporadic cases may occur at any time.

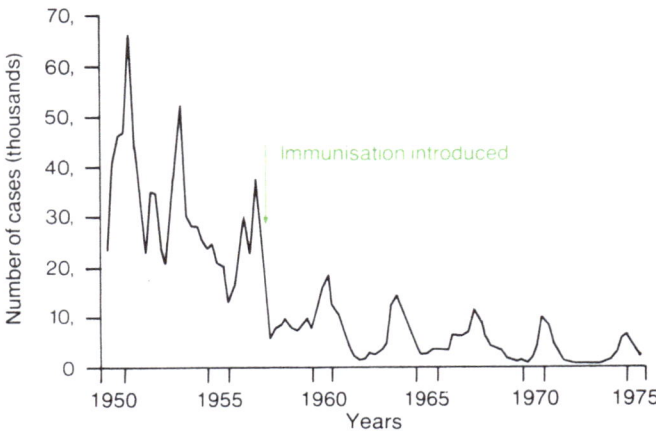

Figure 3. *Quarterly notifications for whooping cough in England and Wales, 1950 to 1975.*

33

Vaccines

Whooping cough vaccines consist of inactivated suspensions of *B. pertussis*. Like other vaccines prepared from whole bacterial cells (e.g. typhoid and cholera), whooping cough vaccines are not comparable in efficacy to the toxoid vaccines (such as those for diphtheria and tetanus) or to virus vaccines. However, although the presently available vaccines may not always prevent pertussis, they do appear to modify the severity of the attack.

The number of cases occurring in immunised children will depend on the efficacy of the vaccine and the proportion of the child population which has been immunised. The higher the percentage of babies vaccinated the greater, proportionally, will be the number of cases occurring in vaccinated individuals. This number will also be greater with less effective vaccines. Thus, if 80 per cent of children in a community are immunised with a 75 per cent effective vaccine, one-fifth of the cases could occur in immunised children. If 100 per cent of children are immunised with a vaccine which is only 20 per cent effective, then 80 per cent of cases could occur in immunised children.

Whooping cough vaccine is commonly given in combination with diphtheria and tetanus toxoids as a triple vaccine (see Chapter 3).

Probably more research has been conducted towards the production of effective vaccines for whooping cough than for any other disease. In the 1940s, field trials carried out in England by the Medical Research Council (MRC) led to the manufacture of what appeared to be satisfactory vaccines. In ten trials where 4,515 children were vaccinated and 4,412 were controls, the average attack rate among siblings with normal home exposure was 18 per cent in the vaccinated and 87 per cent in the unvaccinated group. With other less intimate exposure the attack rates were eight per cent and 38 per cent respectively. One in five of the children in the vaccinated and unvaccinated groups was visited within 24 to 72 hours after each inoculation. In children immunised with vaccines which contained no alum no severe local or general reactions were observed. Several developed a rise in temperature within 24 hours of inoculation and in some the inoculation site was red and swollen for one day to two days. However, in only a few were the reactions such that the mother objected to having the course of immunisation completed. (Where alum-containing vaccines were used, six children developed sterile abscesses.)

Although there were variations in the potency of different batches of vaccines, even from the same source, the success of these trials set the stage for the introduction of whooping cough vaccine as a routine immunisation procedure in Britain.

Most countries which have introduced immunisation against whooping cough seem to have had little or no problem with their immunisation programmes. For example, in the USA cases and consequently deaths from pertussis have declined dramatically with the widespread use of vaccine since the late 1940s with apparently few problems.

Efficacy of Vaccines

Notification is erratic among general practitioners as a whole and inconsistent even for an individual doctor. However, it provides the most useful available index of the community effect of immunisation (Figure 4).

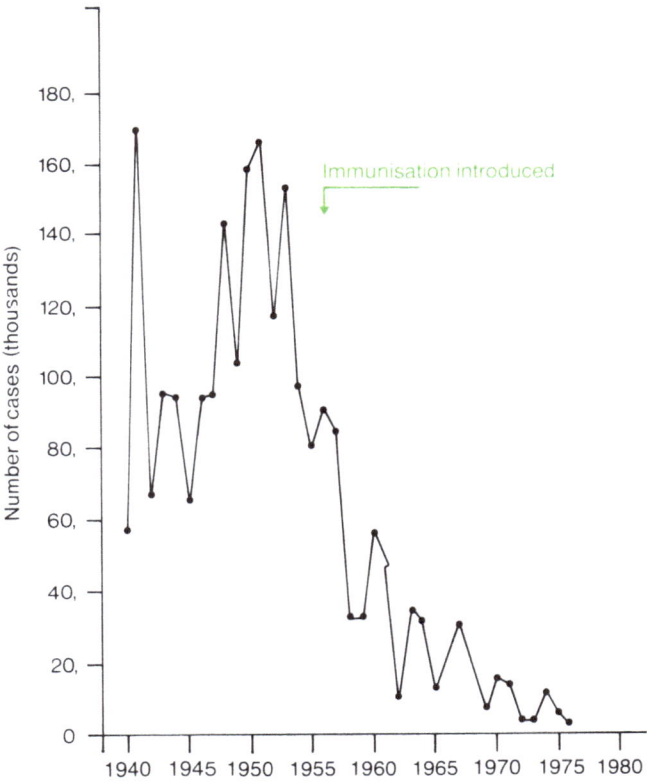

Figure 4. *Whooping cough notifications in England and Wales, 1940 to present.*

Immunisation

Following the introduction of whooping cough vaccine in 1957 in the UK there was about a ten-fold drop in notifications (Figure 5). In spite of reasonably good coverage of vaccine, the subsequent decline in morbidity was not what might have been expected from vaccines, some of which were claimed to give a protection rate of up to 90 per cent in home exposures. Accordingly in the 1960s another field trial was carried out by the Public Health Laboratory Service, and it was discovered that as many as 56 per cent of fully vaccinated children under four years of age developed whooping cough (confirmed bacteriologically), when exposed to pertussis in their homes. This was only a little less than cases in an unvaccinated control group of children and it was concluded that some of the vaccine used before 1966 had an efficacy of only about 20 per cent. Vaccine used in the UK before 1966 had less than the required potency of 4 i.u. and this might account for the apparent vaccine failure. Alternatively, the serotypes of the prevalent strains of *B. pertussis* might have undergone changes and the new serotypes would not be represented in the vaccine. This explanation is not accepted by the majority of experts in Europe or the USA who note that the decline in the incidence of whooping cough which many countries have experienced in

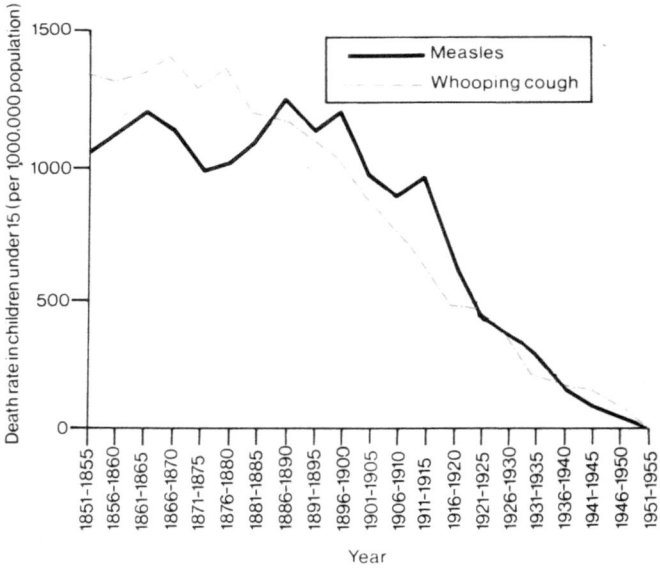

Figure 5. *Decline in deaths from whooping cough and measles (England and Wales).*

the past few years has occurred in spite of using vaccines which did not contain serotypes of the current strains. (When a relatively impotent vaccine was being used in the early and mid-1960s why did notifications not increase proportionately?)

Mortality

For the past century there has been a steady decline in the recorded mortality from all infectious diseases in developed countries. In England and Wales until a few years ago (when measles vaccine became available), the decline in the mortality from whooping cough and that from measles had been very similar for 100 years (see Figure 5). The number of deaths began to fall long before there were vaccines or any effective drugs for their treatment or complications.

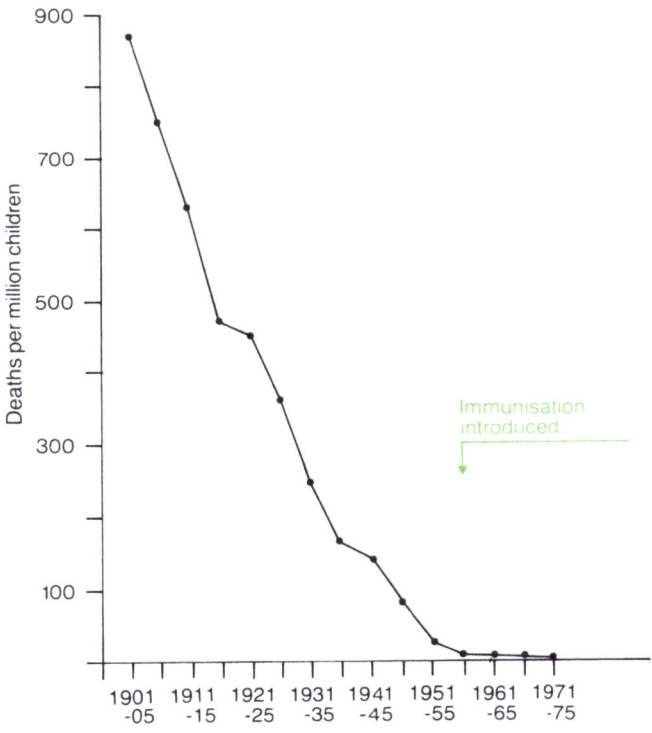

Figure 6. *Deaths from whooping cough per million children under 15 years of age.*

Immunisation

When diphtheria toxoid was introduced the mortality from diphtheria showed an accelerated decline. On the other hand when whooping cough vaccine was introduced no such dramatic drop in mortality was seen but the disease continued its steady decline (see Figures 6 and 7). Vaccine does not appear to have had the influence which might have been expected on the decline of deaths. In previous chapters reference was made to the natural variations over the years of the severity of diphtheria and of scarlet fever. Could the fact that whooping cough has generally become a less fatal and a milder disease in recent years be related to a secular trend rather than to the use of vaccines?

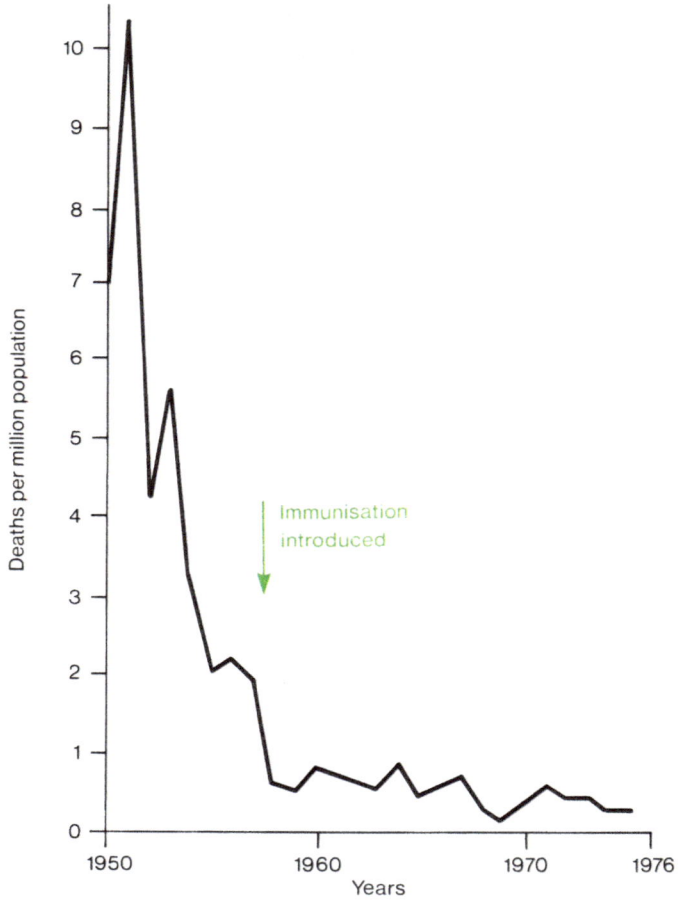

Figure 7. *Whooping cough deaths per million population, England and Wales: 1950 to 1976.*

In the USA approximately 70 per cent of deaths are in children under one year of age. A similar pattern is seen in England and Wales (Table 8). It was suggested many years ago that as far as measles is concerned, anything which tends to postpone the age of attack will tend to make the disease less fatal. This also applies to whooping cough. Deaths from whooping cough have always tended to occur in young children (see Tables 8 and 9). It would seem that the reduction in family size, particularly in poor families, has been an important factor in the reduction of the mortality and in general the mortality from whooping cough has been about twenty times higher in social class V than in social class I. Infection is presumably brought to the family by the young school child. Where there are large families with many small children and babies living in poor, crowded conditions, the disease causes more deaths than among small families living in better conditions.

Reactions

Although reactions to the vaccines used in the MRC trials in the UK in the late 1950s were said to be rare, it appears that they were more

Table 8. Number of deaths from whooping cough (England and Wales) by age (months) 1970 to 1974.

Under 3	3–5	6–11	12 and over	All
26	14	6	7	53

frequent with some vaccines in use in the 1960s. Quite a high proportion of children developed *mild* reactions following immunisation. These minor reactions usually became apparent within a few hours after inoculation and passed off within 12 to 24 hours. The baby became fretful, flushed, feverish and irritable with a painful and swollen arm which could often be relieved with baby aspirin and a cooling lotion such as Lotio calamine. In order to reduce reactions, some doctors have recommended a dose of baby aspirin routinely before immunisation but there is no recorded study of its efficacy in this respect. Major reactions of persistent high pitched screaming, collapse, convulsions and encephalopathy have also been described. The latter is associated with bizarre CNS signs and symptoms and its onset is usually within 24 hours of inoculation. This condition is so rare that the majority of doctors will never see it and if they do it may not be recognized as a complication of vaccination but as indicative of a pre-existing illness. Convulsions and fits which have been recorded as following whooping cough vaccine are so frequent in small babies that they may occur by chance following an immunisation and may not be causally associated. It is not easy to establish an association between an immunisation and a reaction unless it has a characteristic clinical picture and a definite time of onset following immunisation. Preferably there should be a confirmatory laboratory test.

Table 9. Deaths per 1,000 notifications (England and Wales).

Year	Under 1 year	1 to 4 years	5 to 9 years
1944–45	63.7	6.99	1.05
1946–49	42.6	4.07	0.40
1950–53	15.9	1.24	0.12
1954–57	8.8	0.55	0.09
1958–61	5.3	0.46	0.07
1962–65	9.2	0.60	0.04
1966–69	8.7	0.13	—
1970–73	8.2	0.24	0.14

It is well recognized that there is considerable under-reporting of adverse reactions. Controlled prospective studies are required and are at present underway in the UK to try to establish the frequency of convulsions, fits and encephalopathy associated with pertussis vaccine.

Although no published data are as yet available, the frequency of reactions associated with the current vaccines used in the UK appears to be very much less than it was with some of the vaccines in use in the early 1960s. In most other countries of the world the reactions following whooping cough vaccines seem to have been negligible. However, they have caused some concern in Sweden, the Netherlands and in Denmark (where pertussis vaccine is no longer given combined with dip/tet toxoids but as a separate immunisation), and in Hamburg where the vaccine is not at present recommended as a routine procedure.

Contraindications

With all vaccines it appears that reactions can be greatly reduced by observing the contraindications to vaccination. As previously noted no sick child should be immunised. No child who had a severe local or general reaction to a preceding dose should be given a further dose of pertussis vaccine. A history of seizures, convulsions or cerebral irritation in the neonatal period, the presence of any neurological defects or a family history of epilepsy or other diseases of the CNS are also contraindications.

Although allergy has been regarded as a contraindication to immunisation, a considerable body of medical opinion no longer considers this to be so.

Age of Immunisation

The age of immunisation against whooping cough varies from country to country (see Chapters 2 and 14). There is very little evidence that the vaccine is effective if given in the first few months of life (certainly very small babies are less efficient in their agglutinin responses than older ones). As previously noted, one study found that reactions to whooping cough vaccine were twenty times greater in babies under six months than in older ones. Quite apart from the possible danger of more frequent reactions in smaller babies, mothers are nowadays loath to complete courses if their babies have been even mildly upset following an injection.

The schedules recommended in the USA and UK of starting immunisation at from two to six months can give little direct protection to small babies. However, the objective is the control of the disease in toddlers and preschool children where there is the greatest morbidity, thus reducing the chance of the infection being brought back into the family and spreading to small babies.

It might be possible to control an outbreak in some countries by a 'fire brigade action'. With an increased incidence of cases in any district, small babies might be immunised immediately with a course of three injections of pertussis vaccine at two- to three-week intervals. The extent of such outbreak control programmes would depend on the local situation and it would have to be followed up later by routine immunisation with triple vaccine. In general, immunisation of babies under one month is not recommended as a routine measure.

41

6. Smallpox

Up to about 30 years ago the USA had several thousand cases of smallpox each year. The large number of cases in the USA early in this century was generally attributed to the variation in the vaccination requirements of the 50 states, and it was claimed, without good evidence, that the frequency of smallpox varied inversely with the rigidity of the State's vaccination requirement. No importation of smallpox into the USA has occurred since 1949. Although there have been many importations of smallpox into the UK since the disease became non-endemic in 1935, all of these importations were readily controlled, in spite of the fact that the herd immunity in recent years has only been about 10 per cent, for the number of infant vaccinations had been steadily declining since the beginning of the century when about three-quarters of the infants in Britain were vaccinated.

The Vaccination Act of 1905 made conscientious objection to what was at that time a compulsory procedure much easier. By 1914 the number of children vaccinated was below 50 per cent. The decline continued over the years and compulsory vaccination of infants ended with the introduction of the National Health Service in 1946. Nevertheless, the majority of physicians and the DHSS recommended that infant vaccination should be assiduously pursued although between 1951 and 1970 there had been at least 101 deaths from vaccination and only 37 deaths from smallpox. In 1972 there was a sudden change in policy and routine smallpox vaccination was no longer recommended in the UK. A similar policy change by the United States Public Health Services occurred in 1971. What had led to these about-turns in national policies?

Two things had happened. First, it was recognized that there were many more complications following vaccination than had been generally realized, and second the World Health Organization's global programme of smallpox eradication, started in 1967, was proceeding successfully.

Before looking in detail at the findings which have led to the abandonment of routine infant vaccination in the UK, the USA and Canada, one or two facts about the disease and its epidemiology should be recalled.

Epidemiology and Natural History

Although many species of animals and birds have their own pox viruses, no reservoir of smallpox virus other than man has been discovered.

There are two types of smallpox: variola major which had a case mortality rate of 30 to 50 per cent and variola minor, which has a less than 1 per cent case fatality rate. Smallpox was endemic in Britain and America for centuries and before vaccination most people hoped to catch the disease in milder form in order to prevent an attack of this usually severe, disfiguring and highly fatal condition. So dreaded was the disease in prevaccination days, that mothers would even expose their babies to infection in the hope that if they acquired smallpox when they were young it would be mild. This old wives' tale could be explained by the disease being modified by the protective effect of maternally transmitted gamma globulin. The probability of acquiring smallpox in the 19th century was so great that people were prepared to accept the risk of dying from the intentional inoculation of smallpox (variolation) rather than risk catching the disease. This prophylactic 'ingrafting' or variolation had been practised for centuries in many eastern countries before it was introduced into Europe towards the end of the 17th century. It appears that the mortality from variolation was about ten times less than that of a natural infection with variola major. It is possible that virus which has multiplied in the skin is less virulent than virus from the nasopharynx which is the usual source of virus in the transmission of smallpox. Furthermore, the abnormal site of virus invasion, namely the skin, may have been responsible for a milder outcome of the infection.

Although endemic smallpox lingered in Britain as variola minor until 1935, the last major epidemics of variola major occurred at the beginning of this century.

Smallpox is usually transmitted by direct face to face contact or by contact with infected clothing, bedding or other materials. The disease is not infectious during the incubation period, but with the onset of fever before the appearance of the skin rash the patient is highly infectious

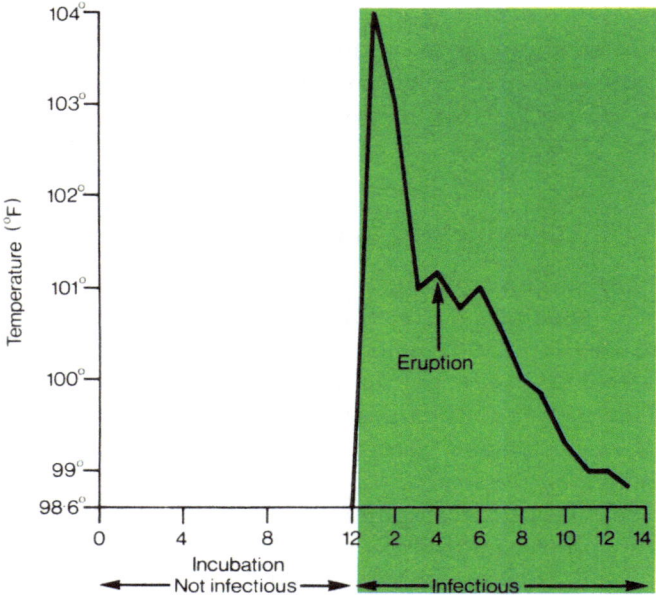

Figure 8. *Infectious and non-infectious periods.*

(Figure 8). In the classic infection patients are usually confined to bed in the first few days of the disease and are not a danger to the community except their family contacts. Patients with the disease modified by previous vaccination may sometimes be more of a problem in spreading the disease.

History of Vaccination

The belief of the apocryphal milk maid who is said to have remarked 'I cannot take small pox for I have had cow pox' was fairly widely accepted in parts of England in the middle of the 18th century. Although Benjamin Jesty, a Dorset farmer, was honoured as the first vaccinator he was not the first person to have discovered that the inoculation of cow pox prevented not only an attack of cow pox but also of smallpox. Jesty scratched the arms of his wife and two sons with material from cow pox lesions from the udders of cows. The Jesty family were all subsequently resistant to natural infection with smallpox and the two boys resisted a challenge of smallpox by inoculation some years later. Edward Jenner's most important scientific contribution was his successful transfer of cow pox from person to person. Successful virus passage and vaccinations with lymph passed from person to person were recorded in *An Inquiry into the Causes and Effect of the Variolate Vaccinae, a disease discovered in some of the Western Counties of England, particularly Gloucestershire, and known by the name of Cow Pox*, which was published in 1798.

In 1840 variolation was made illegal following the introduction of the first Vaccination Act, and smallpox gradually disappeared from the UK. Although the introduction of vaccination with 'humanized' lymph had considerable opposition, the vaccination of infants was made compulsory in 1853 and enforced in 1871 in the UK and 1855 and 1872 in the USA. Following the introduction of vaccination the decline of the disease was not dramatic. Better social conditions, the control of vagrants, the establishment of workhouses, the setting up of smallpox hospitals and the surveillance and recording of disease all played a highly important part in its control, as did the cessation of variolation, which eliminated a source of virus.

The Vaccine

At the beginning of this century, the preparation of lymph in the skin of calves became approved. This led to the use of standardized lymph to which glycerine was added to reduce the bacterial contamination. Humanized lymph, with its attendant dangers of bacterial contamination and the accidental transfer of smallpox, was soon given up.

The origins of the various strains of calf lymph vaccinia virus are uncertain. Vaccinia virus differs from both cow pox and smallpox viruses. Some strains of vaccinia may be mutants of either cow pox or smallpox virus. One of the commonly used strains is said to have been derived from a mild case of smallpox in the Franco-Prussian War. Alternatively, vaccinia could represent a stable recombinant of cow pox and smallpox viruses.

Today, sheep are used instead of calves as vaccinifers in many laboratories with an occasional passage of stock virus in rabbit or man in order to maintain high titre vaccines.

In the preparation of the vaccine lymph the animal's belly and thorax are washed and shaved and virus is applied with a scalpel in a series of parallel superficial incisions. After about four days the vesicles which have developed are scraped off and the resulting pulp is ground up with glycerol and stored at $-10°$ C to reduce the bacterial content. Other methods have been introduced in order to produce bacteriologically

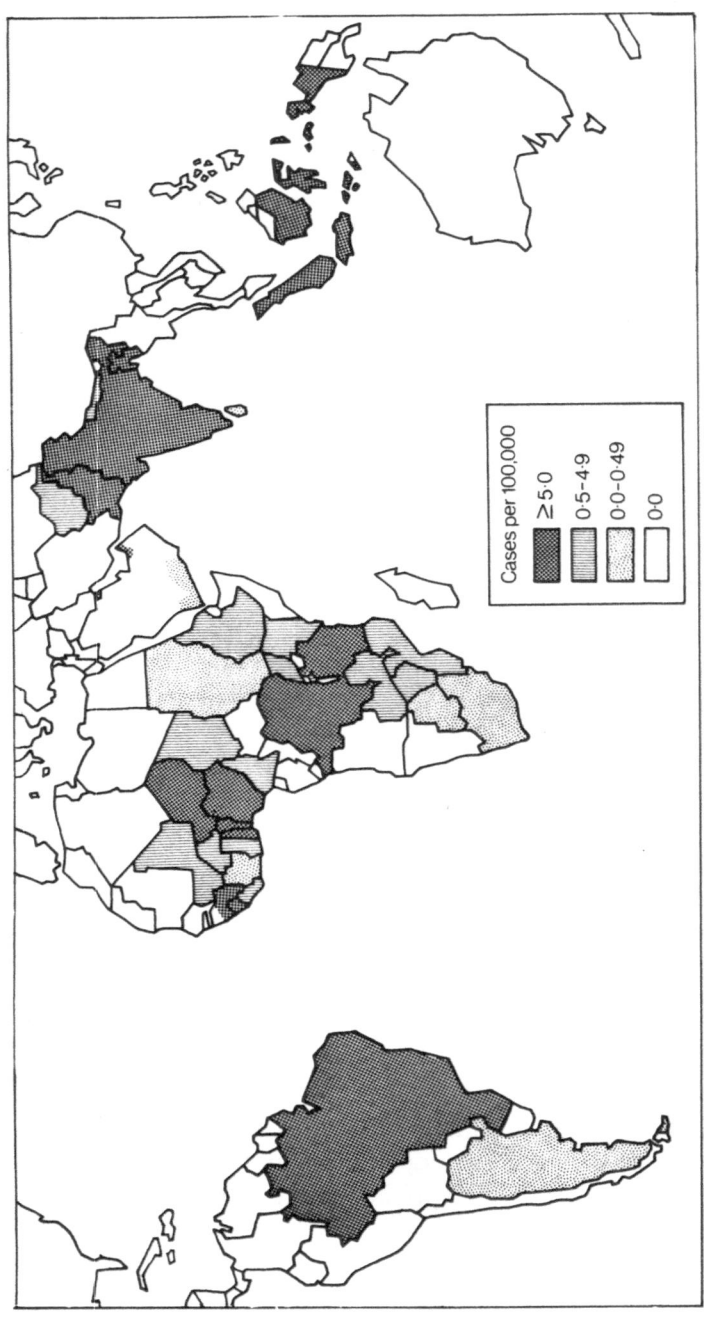

Figure 9. *Smallpox cases per 100,000 inhabitants: 1967.*

sterile standard preparations of lymph including the growth of virus in chick-embryos or in tissue cultures.

The availability of refrigeration to prevent deterioration on storage played an important part in maintaining the efficacy of vaccinia virus. The development of stable freeze-dried vaccine made global eradication of smallpox a practical proposition in a relatively short time.

'Global Eradication'

In 1967 there were probably about 2,500,000 cases of smallpox in the world arising in 42 countries. Thirty of these had endemic smallpox and 12 had imported the disease (Figure 9). By 1973 only four countries—Ethiopia, India, Bangladesh and Pakistan—were considered to be endemic areas (Figure 10). By that year smallpox had been eradicated from South America as indicated by the absence of any cases following two years of active surveillance after the discovery of the last known case. Subsequently eradication has been certified in Indonesia in 1974 and in Afghanistan, Pakistan and Western Africa in 1976. At that time Ethiopia remained the only endemic country in the world. By early 1978 smallpox has become limited to a few cases of variola minor among Somali nomads along the Somalia/Ethiopia/Kenya borders, and hopefully by the end of 1978 there will be global eradication.

Technique of Vaccination

The development of the bifurcated needle has played a most valuable part in community vaccination programmes in the developing countries of the world.

For the elective vaccination of travellers and for outbreak control (if it is ever again required) those with little or no experience of vaccination and those who have not reassessed their technique in recent years should consult the latest edition of the *Memorandum on Vaccination against Smallpox* (1974), HMSO or the Report of the American Public Health Association on Control of Communicable Diseases in Man, 12th edition, edited by A. S. Benenson (1975).

Vaccination is best done on the arm, inside the mid-line at the junction of the middle and upper thirds. Any scarring will be least noticeable at this site and the vaccinial lesion will be best protected. Any preparation of the site is contraindicated and no disinfectant should be used. If the area is dirty it may be cleaned with soap and water.

A minimum trauma technique should be used. For primary vac-

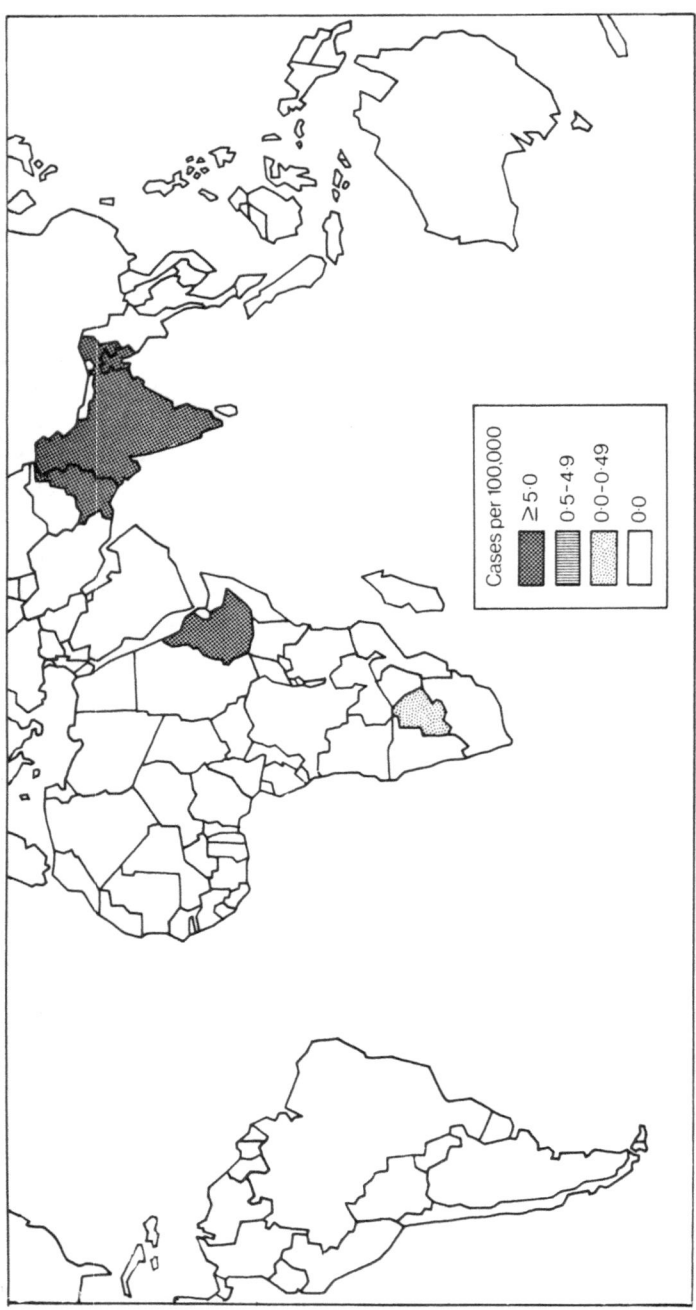

Figure 10. *Smallpox cases per 100,000 inhabitants (estimated): 1973.*

cination, a single scratch of about one-sixth to one-eighth of an inch long is sufficient. If the multiple puncture technique is used no more than 10 pressures should be made within an area of one-eighth inch diameter. For revaccination a single scratch of about one-quarter inch or 30 pressures should be given. In outbreak control, vaccination of contacts should consist of two scarifications about one-quarter to one-half of an inch long or 30 pressures over two areas about one inch apart.

A little bleeding seems to be of no great importance but should be avoided if possible. Excess vaccine should be wiped off after about 30 seconds with a sterile gauze and the remainder allowed to dry. No dressing is usually required and Elastoplast and occlusive dressings are contraindicated. A light gauze bandage may be put around the arm or a square of gauze pinned inside the shirt or blouse covering the area. If the vaccine is in plastic tubing the scissors used to snip the plastic should be boiled after use and preferably a pair of scissors should be kept solely for this purpose. Vaccinators should never forget the possibility of accidental vaccination of themselves or other patients.

About seven days after vaccination the site should be inspected. The result should be recorded as either a 'major' or 'equivocal' reaction (one no longer talks about 'reactions of immunity' etc. which usually only indicate protein sensitivity).

A major reaction after primary vaccination is a typical Jennerian vesicle. After revaccination a vesicle or pustule, or an area of definite palpable induration or congestion surrounding a central lesion, which may be a scab or an ulcer, constitute a major reaction.

If a major reaction has not been obtained one week after the vaccination, the procedure should be repeated. If no reaction is obtained after repeated revaccinations, 'no local reaction to repeated vaccinations' should be recorded on the certificate.

Contraindications

The contraindications (except for outbreak control for which there are no absolute contraindications) are:

1. A history of, or the presence of eczema in the vaccinee or in any contact of a vaccinated person. Such individuals should be kept away from any recently vaccinated person for three weeks.

2. Hypogammaglobulinaemia or other immunological abnormalities.

3. Lymphoma, leukaemia or other tumours of the reticuloendothelial system.

4. Corticosteroid or other immunosuppressive therapy or radiotherapy.

5. Septic skin conditions, exposure to infectious diseases and failure of an infant to thrive.

6. Pregnancy is a contraindication to immunisation with all live virus vaccines. In a pregnancy in which there has been no interference, the risk of fetal vaccinia appears to be infinitesimally small and there is no evidence that vaccinia is teratogenic. Vaccination of a woman who is subsequently found to be pregnant is not an indication for termination of the pregnancy.

While there is no absolute contraindication to the vaccination of contacts of smallpox cases, antivaccinial immunoglobulin should also be given to all family contacts. If a patient has a contraindication to vaccination and requires vaccination for foreign travel 750 mg of antivaccinial gamma globulin should be given into the opposite arm at the same time as vaccination. In the USA the equivalent is vaccinia immune globulin (VIG), 0.3 ml per kg. In England and Wales this may be obtained through one of the PHLS laboratories: in the USA it may be obtained commercially or from one of the consultants listed by the regional blood centres of the Red Cross.

Complications of Vaccination

Table 10 shows the number and types of complications which occurred in the UK between 1951 and 1970 following smallpox vaccination. All of these complications, except postvaccinial encephalitis, could probably have been greatly reduced by paying attention to the contraindications to vaccination and nòt vaccinating babies in the first year of life where complication rates are highest. With the abandonment of routine immunisation these complications are now largely of academic and historic interest in Britain and North America.

The commonest complication and the one for which no contraindication to vaccination or prevention is recognized is postvaccinial encephalitis. Although accurate denominators are difficult to estimate, Table 11 demonstrates that there is no evidence to support the contention that postvaccinial encephalitis is commoner in adults than in children. This also applies to the other complications.

Abandonment of Infant Vaccination

The arguments for the abandonment of routine infant vaccination in

Britain and the USA centred mainly around the frequency of complications of vaccination and the fact that with the global control of smallpox the chance of importations and spread from them was decreasing.

Some argued that those countries which stopped infant vaccination would be wide open to epidemics if and when smallpox was imported or 'escaped'. They forgot that the UK, with a vaccine acceptance rate of only about 30 to 40 per cent, had been susceptible to the spread from importations for years. Smallpox does not spread very quickly, and infant vaccination (contrary to the opinion of Jenner) does not give life-long protection. Furthermore, the herd immunity in the UK in the 1960s was only about 5 to 10 per cent. In any event, small children were not at high risk of being infected following importations, and experience in recent years in the UK and in the rest of Europe has incriminated the hospital as the setting for most outbreaks of smallpox. Until global eradication occurs there is always a possibility of importing smallpox but compared with 10 years ago the risk of doing so is now virtually negligible.

A final objection to the abandonment of infant vaccination came from those who said that complications of vaccination are commoner in adults than in children.

Selective Epidemiological Control

Between 1951 and 1970 there were 13 importations into the UK. All of these were successfully limited by selective epidemiological control methods. There is no place for mass vaccination in the control of an outbreak, for it takes up the time of those carrying out selective epidemiological control, leads to bad work by improvised staff and kills people who need never have been vaccinated.

The selective epidemiological control technique involves quarantining of patients and prompt tracing, vaccination and surveillance of known or probable contacts. Vaccination on the first day or so after contact prevents infection, and if it is done within the first few days after contact the disease will often be modified. The reason for this protective effect of vaccination is that immunity to vaccinia virus develops more rapidly than to variola major virus.

Since contacts are not infectious during the incubation period (Figure 8) they can be kept under surveillance after vaccination. Some argue that outbreak control can hardly prove to be as effective in an unvac-

Table 10. The number and types of complications which occurred following smallpox vaccination in the UK between 1951 and 1970.

Complications	No.
Postvaccinial encephalitis	40
Contact eczema vaccinatum	16
Vaccinia gangrenosa	13
Eczema vaccinatum	11
Benign generalized vaccinia	2
Others	19

Table 11. Complications and deaths from postvaccinial encephalitis in England and Wales between 1951 and 1970. (Rates per million vaccinations.)

Age in years	Approx. numbers of vaccinations (thousands)	Complications		Deaths	
		No.	Rate	No.	Rate
Under 1	3,734	51	13.7	20	5.4
1–4	3,733	32	8.6	8	2.1
5–15	2,689	19	7.0	2	0.7
15 plus	5,509	45	8.2	6	0.9

cinated community as in a partially vaccinated community. However, outbreaks in England this century have never been related to the proportion of vaccinated persons, which has varied from 2 to 75 per cent in the communities involved. The increased success of the WHO eradication programme in recent years has not been the result of stepping up indiscriminate mass vaccination, but of the application of selective epidemiological control methods based on searching for cases, and the vaccination and surveillance of their contacts. Indeed, smallpox was eradicated from Mali and from Sierra Leone which had the highest rates in the world, when only 51 and 66 per cent respectively of the population had been vaccinated.

Escapes

With the global eradication of human-to-human transmission and the failure to discover any non-human links in the chain of infection, the only possible remaining reservoirs of smallpox are laboratory stocks of virus. Although only two instances of laboratory-acquired infections have been described, the outbreak of four cases in London in 1973 emphasizes the possible risk. Accordingly WHO are encouraging laboratories not requiring variola virus for research purposes to destroy their stocks of the virus. Also, a register is being kept of those laboratories holding such stocks.

The Future

The world should be certified free of smallpox by 1980 and the first, and for many years the only, infectious disease to be controlled by immunisation will have been eradicated. Most countries will eventually give up routine smallpox immunisation but *when* this occurs will depend on the efficacy of their surveillance programmes. It is likely that most countries will retain adequate stocks of smallpox vaccine so that if changes in the epidemiology of smallpox occur, alterations in the vaccination policy can be made overnight.

7. Poliomyelitis

Although poliomyelitis has been endemic for centuries it was not till about 80 years ago that it first became an epidemic disease, first in Scandinavia and later in the USA where regular epidemics occurred from the early 1900s until the mid-1950s when immunisation was introduced.

In the UK, about the beginning of this century, as in the earlier outbreaks in the USA, poliomyelitis was essentially 'infantile paralysis' and in one of these epidemics in Bristol in 1909, 80 per cent of the 37 paralytic cases occurred in children under three years of age. In the 1900s there were small scattered outbreaks in various parts of Britain until after the Second World War, but none of them was on the scale of the epidemics occurring at that time in Scandinavia or the USA. Then in 1947 there was a sudden increase in incidence and the total number of cases rose to 7,776 compared with the previous highest figure of 1,489 in 1938. Over the years, there was also a change in age of attack. Between 1912 (when the disease became notifiable) and 1920 about 65 per cent of cases were in the 0 to 4 year old group and 30 per cent in the 5 to 14 year olds. In contrast, between 1942 and 1950 one third of cases were in the 0 to 4, 5 to 14, and over 15 age groups.

Why there was a sudden increase in 1947 remains a mystery. Yearly epidemics of varying severity continued until 1958 when vaccine was introduced. After this, what Simon Flexner called 'this saddest of diseases', which left many persons permanently paralysed, appears to have become a thing of the past in North America and much of Europe. However, constant vigilance is still required.

This shift from endemic to epidemic poliomyelitis has followed this characteristic pattern in all countries and it appears that the incidence of poliomyelitis bears an inverse relation to infant mortality. When the number of deaths per 1,000 live births falls below 75, poliomyelitis changes from an endemic to an epidemic disease. The implication of these findings for developing countries is obvious.

Natural History

Polioviruses enter the body by the mouth and replicate in the pharynx, intestine and lymph nodes (Figure 11).

The virus may get into the blood (depending on the strain) and the viraemia which may result in a number of individuals can lead to invasion of the CNS with subsequent destruction of neurones leading to paralysis. However, paralysis is a rare outcome, and the vast majority of infections with polioviruses go unrecognized. Depending on the strain of the virus and the susceptibility of population, there may be from about 100 to 1,000 subclinical infections to each clinical case.

There are three types of poliovirus: Types 1, 2 and 3. Type 1 has been responsible for about 60 per cent of all paralytic cases in the northern hemisphere. Although there are minor antigenic differences between various strains, all have similar characteristics and the immunity to each of them is essentially type-specific.

The viruses are transmitted from person to person by the faecal–oral route, but no one knows if oropharyngeal virus or faecal virus is the more important in the spread of disease.

Vaccines

There are two types of poliovirus vaccines, namely inactivated poliovirus vaccines (IPV) and live attenuated oral poliovirus vaccines (OPV).

While only the latter is now in routine use in the UK and USA, it must not be forgotten that poliomyelitis was nearly completely controlled in the UK by IPV (Figure 12). It is still the *only* type of vaccine in use in Sweden, Finland and the Netherlands, and some IPV is also used in Canada. Poliomyelitis has been eradicated from Sweden, and in the Netherlands the disease has occurred only rarely since the introduction of inactivated vaccines (essentially in communities which have resisted immunisation on religious grounds).

Inactivated Poliovirus Vaccines (IPV)

These are manufactured by growing each type of poliovirus in tissue culture and inactivating the virus-rich tissue culture fluids with for-

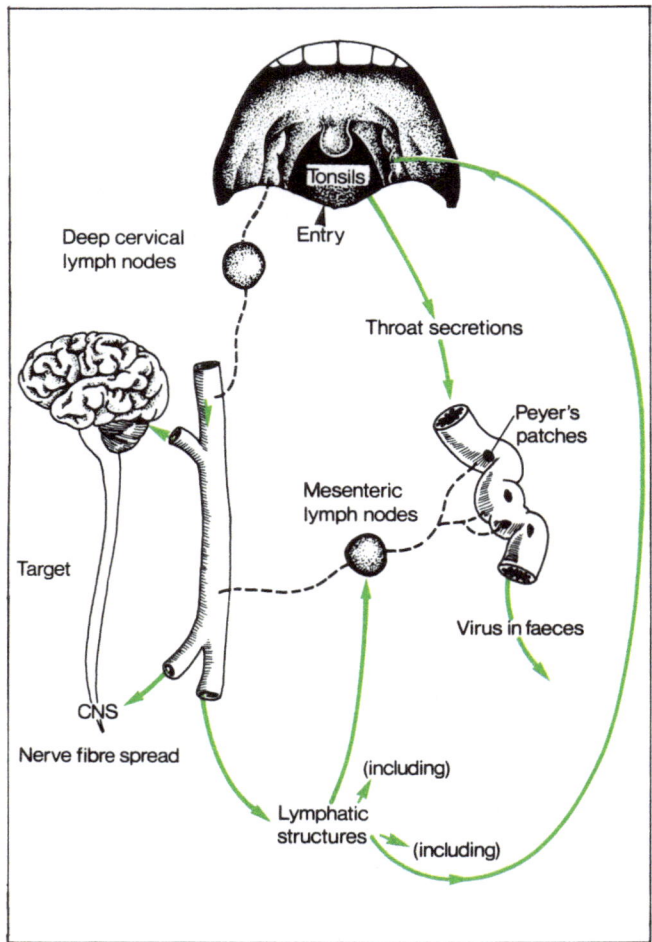

Figure 11. *Pathogenesis of poliomyelitis.*

malin. After filtration, the three types of inactivated viruses are blended in the required proportions.

When potent vaccines are used and given at properly spaced intervals, IPV stimulates high levels of neutralizing antibody. As with other inactivated antigens, primary immunisation with IPV sensitizes the body to react with a secondary response when the antigen is encountered either as an infection or when the individual is given a booster inoculation.

The immunity induced by IPV is essentially due to circulating antibodies which neutralize the virus and prevent its spread from the

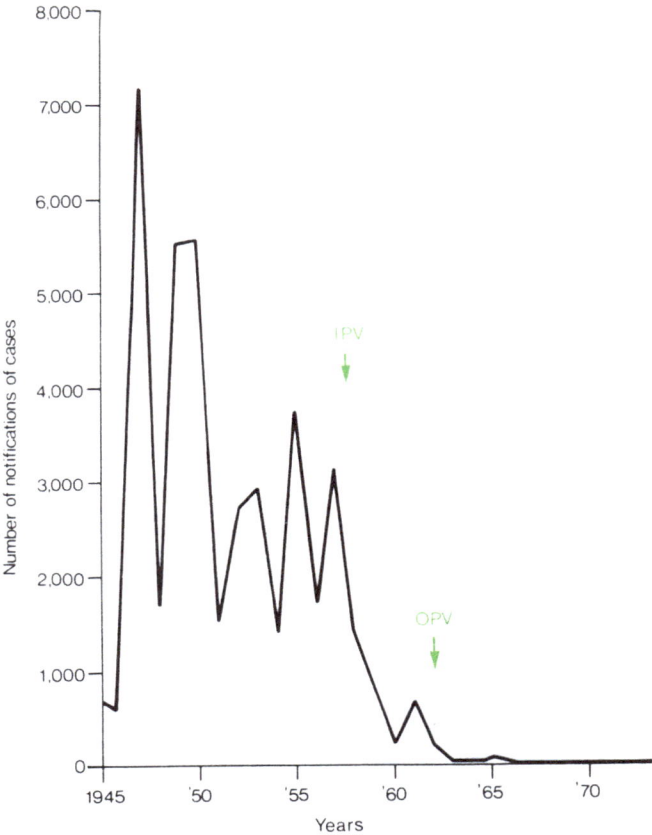

Figure 12. *Notifications of paralytic poliomyelitis (England and Wales).*

alimentary canal to the CNS. The levels of antibody which can be attained by IPV are higher than those induced by OPV and it seems that this serological immunity is as durable, if not more so, than that following OPV.

Indeed, the antibody levels with potent IPV approximate the maximum obtainable, and are subsequently more readily boosted by a single injection of IPV than by a dose of OPV.

Efficacy

Although the routine introduction of IPV on a wide scale in 1959 had a dramatic effect on paralytic poliomyelitis in Europe and North America, there was a small rise in the incidence and deaths from poliomyelitis in 1960 and 1961 (Figure 12).

This rise was explained by the relatively poor antigenicity of the Type 1 component. In early vaccines this was the least effective, though Type 1 was the most frequently paralytic virus.

Because of the high efficacy of the Type 2 component in the vaccine, Type 2 virus practically disappeared from those countries with effective immunisation programmes. However, no effort was made to improve IPV at that time, for it was generally considered that a better vaccine (OPV) was just around the corner.

Nevertheless, with a relatively impotent IPV, poliomyelitis was almost eliminated. The potency of the IPV which is available today is about ten times greater than that of vaccines produced in the late 1950s.

Herd Immunity

It is not always appreciated that IPV has a profound epidemiological effect in preventing the spread of polioviruses. In Sweden, where only IVP has been used routinely, both poliomyelitis and polioviruses have disappeared.

Trials in Belfast showed that when live poliovirus was given to individuals immunised with IPV, not only could virus not be recovered from the oropharynx but faecal excretion of virus was greatly reduced. It was, therefore, unlikely that such persons would transmit the disease if they were infected.

Reactions

In the early days of IPV it was found that live virus was present in some batches of vaccine which produced paralytic poliomyelitis in some inoculated children and their contacts. However, since 1962, with improved manufacturing and safety-testing techniques, IPV has been one of the safest vaccines available.

Side-effects are rare: some IPV contains traces of streptomycin and neomycin and the possibility of reactions in sensitive individuals must be remembered.

In general, with millions of doses only a few complications like the Guillain–Barré syndrome, encephalopathy and convulsions have been recorded. Since purified vaccines were introduced, adverse effects seem to have been even less frequent.

Use of IPV

While IPV is not used routinely, it is available for individuals in whom OPV is contraindicated. These include pregnant women, patients undergoing corticosteroid therapy or those with intestinal dysfunction.

Dip/tet/polio may be used as an alternative to dip/tet and OPV at school entry, and, as noted, IPV more regularly boosts circulating antibody than a single dose of OPV.

IPV has been combined with dip/tet/polio as a quadruple vaccine, and is used in some parts of Canada (in the schedule outlined in Table 12) and in Holland.

Oral Poliovaccine

This is recommended at present for routine use in most countries. The vaccine consists of attenuated strains of each of the three types of poliovirus grown in monkey kidney tissue culture. The vaccine strains have been selected for their lack of neurovirulence when the viruses are injected intraspinally or intracerebrally into monkeys.

Types 1, 2 and 3 attenuated strains have been given separately as monovalent vaccines but for administrative convenience all three types of vaccine are usually given together as a trivalent preparation. The number of virus particles contained in a single dose of trivalent vaccine is usually about 10^6 for Type 1, 10^5 for Type 2 and $10^{5.5}$ for Type 3.

Action of OPV

OPV viruses, like wild polioviruses, multiply in the throat and in the intestine. They stimulate not only circulating antibodies (IgM and IgG) but also IgA, which prevents infection of the intestinal canal.

The immunity with OPV is dependent on replication of the viruses in the gut: if the vaccine virus does not multiply the individual will not become immunised.

One enteric virus can interfere with the replication of another. When trivalent vaccine is fed, to begin with only one of the virus types will colonize the gut and multiply and stimulate immunity (both local and humoral) to that type. One of the other types in the vaccine may remain in the gut and take over when the first colonizing type has ceased to replicate, and so immunity to two types could follow a dose of trivalent OPV. (I have no experience of a successful 'take' of all three types following a single dose of vaccine.)

If the vaccine was given to an individual who, for example, was immune to Type 2 virus as a result of natural Type 2 infection, the Type

Table 12. Recommended schedule for infants and children, using quadruple vaccine, as in Canada.

Age	Immunisation
2 months	Dip/pert/tet/polio (quad)
4 months	Dip/pert/tet/polio (quad)
6 months	Dip/pert/tet/polio (quad)
1 year	Measles vaccine
	Rubella vaccine[1]
$1\frac{1}{2}$ years	Dip/pert/tet/polio (quad)
4 to 6 years	Dip/pert/tet/polio (quad)
11 to 12 years (females only)	Rubella vaccine[1]
14 to 16 years	Dip/tet/polio

[1] At or after 1 year to infants of both sexes or at 12 years to prepubertal girls.

2 vaccine virus would not replicate. However, one or both of the other types could infect and immunise. All sorts of combinations of success or failure to immunise against any one type can occur when oral vaccines are given, for polioviruses like other enteric viruses interfere with each other.

Thus, if a child is carrying an enteric virus, e.g. an Echo or Coxsackie virus—many of which give subclinical infections—then again there may be interference with the vaccine 'take' when OPV is given.

Schedule of Immunisation

OPV does not readily colonize the guts of small babies. It is usually given at the same time as dip/tet/pert, i.e. the first dose at three to six months of age, the second six weeks later, and the third six months later. A reinforcing dose should be given at school entry and another one at school leaving.

Particular attention should be given to immunising immigrant families who may have come from countries with no routine poliomyelitis immunisation programme. Indeed at the present time in several European countries the majority of the cases of poliomyelitis in children involve the families of migrant workers.

In addition to routine immunisation of babies (see schedule, Chapter 2) attention should be paid to immunising young adults who may have escaped immunisation in childhood and consider themselves too old for immunisation. With the disappearance of wild viruses, they could possibly also have escaped a natural immunising infection. Apart from giving a course of vaccine to any young adult who has not been immunised as a baby, boosters should be given to all travellers to countries outside Northern Europe, North America, Australia and New Zealand.

Outbreak Control

Presumably the interference effect of OPV comes into play before the development of protective levels of neutralizing antibody.

This interference phenomenon can be used to control an outbreak. Thus, if a case of poliomyelitis occurs, all contacts, e.g. in school, play area and street, should immediately be given a dose of OPV, regardless of previous history of immunisation. Protection will depend on local conditions, but this 'fire brigade' action should limit the spread of wild strains because of interference induced by the attenuated vaccine viruses.

How interference works is not certain, but presumably the attenuated vaccine virus colonizes the gut and prevents the epidemic strain from attaching to cell receptors.

In the USA poliomyelitis is considered to be epidemic (or potentially epidemic) when there are two or more cases caused by the same type of virus during a four-week period in a defined population. Under these circumstances all persons six weeks of age or older who have not previously received a complete course of OPV should be immunised.

Safety of OPV

Live virus vaccines carry more potential hazards than IPV. In the first place, there are the problems of excluding extraneous agents, mainly those from the monkey kidneys, used in manufacture.

Another aspect of safety is the possibility of the attenuated virus becoming less attenuated on replication in the human gut. Although this danger is much less than had been anticipated, it must be kept in mind not only as a risk to vaccinees but also to their contacts.

The overall risk of paralytic poliomyelitis associated with OPV is of the order of one to three per million doses but this figure relates to communities with a variable proportion of naturally immune individuals. The exact risk in a susceptible population is unknown: it appears to be greater with Type 2 and Type 3 than with Type 1 vaccine.

Because of the possible risk to contacts, when vaccine is being given to the baby of young parents it is important that they should be offered vaccine at the same time, for parents have been paralysed from the progeny of vaccine virus from their own babies. Also, babies who have recently received vaccine should not be put in contact with non-immunised infants. (There is presumptive evidence that one who had been put in the same pram as a recently vaccinated baby contracted a paralytic infection.)

Since the introduction of poliovirus vaccines the UK Public Health Laboratory Service and the CDC (now the Infectious Disease Centre) in Atlanta, Georgia, have carried out surveillance of all cases of poliomyelitis. Vaccine viruses have certain growth characteristics in the laboratory and it is sometimes possible to identify viruses as having the properties of a 'wild virus' or of a 'vaccine virus'. In the UK, of 163 strains isolated in 1972, only 10 had the characteristics of 'wild' viruses. However, it is difficult to decide whether or not a strain recovered from a paralytic or non-paralytic case is vaccine-derived, for very occasionally vaccine viruses may develop the paralytic properties of 'wild' strains. While some may retain their markers, others may lose them and appear to be 'wild' viruses.

Most cases of poliomyelitis in developed countries in the past few years have occurred in unvaccinated individuals. Several of them have been importations by visitors from endemic areas.

Efficacy of OPV

Paralytic and non-paralytic poliomyelitis has virtually disappeared from all countries where there has been good coverage with OPV (as with potent IPV) (Figure 13).

Now that poliomyelitis is rarely found in the UK and USA, is it necessary to immunise against it? The answer is an emphatic *Yes*, for there is still much poliomyelitis throughout the world. While poliomyelitis has tended to disappear from countries with effective immunisation programmes, notifications have increased in some less fortunate developing countries (Figure 14). Poliovirus could be imported 'silently' from many parts of the world and could spread in a poorly immunised community. Failure to maintain effective immunisation programmes in developed countries could lead to a return to an epidemic situation.

It is important to realize that a 75 per cent immunisation rate in children is not enough. We should be attempting to achieve near 100 per cent acceptance rate for both primary immunisations and boosters at school entry and school leaving.

Efficacy must be continuously monitored. Recent studies in places as far apart as Glasgow and Ivanjua in Serbia (where programmes have been carried out with OPV) have indicated some gaps in immunity in school children and young adults. These studies do not support the belief that attenuated strains of OPV will necessarily give lifelong

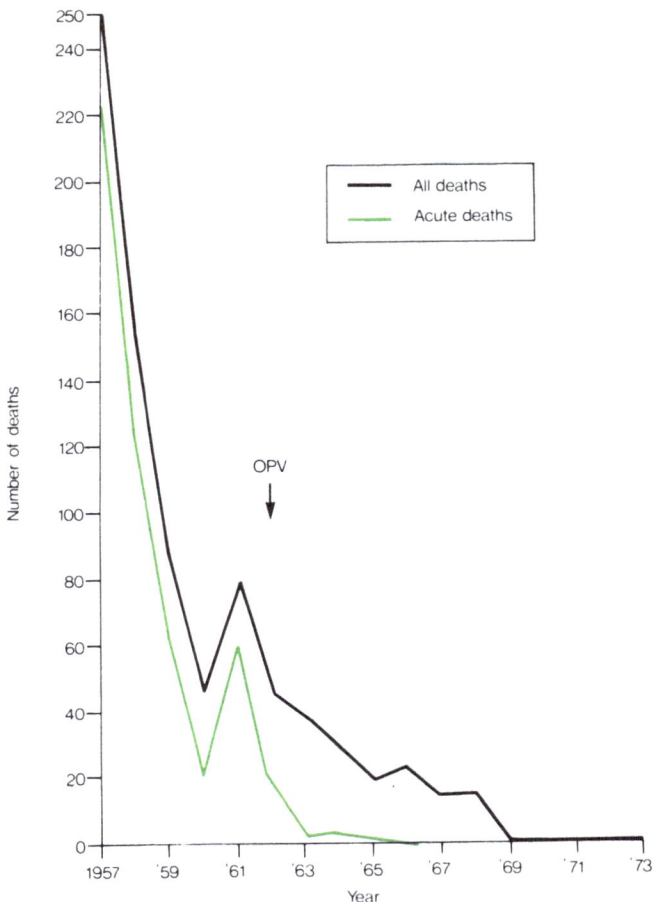

Figure 13. *Deaths from poliomyelitis in the past 16 years (England and Wales).*

immunity. It may be that vaccine strains are less antigenic than 'wild' ones or that repeated experiences with vaccine-type viruses may be necessary, now that the boosting effect of 'wild' strains has virtually disappeared from some countries. Boosters with vaccine *in addition* to those at school entry and school leaving may be required.

Storage of Vaccine

OPV is stored in bulk at −20° C and remains viable for at least six months. After issue from the deep freeze, like all other vaccines it should be held at about +4° C.

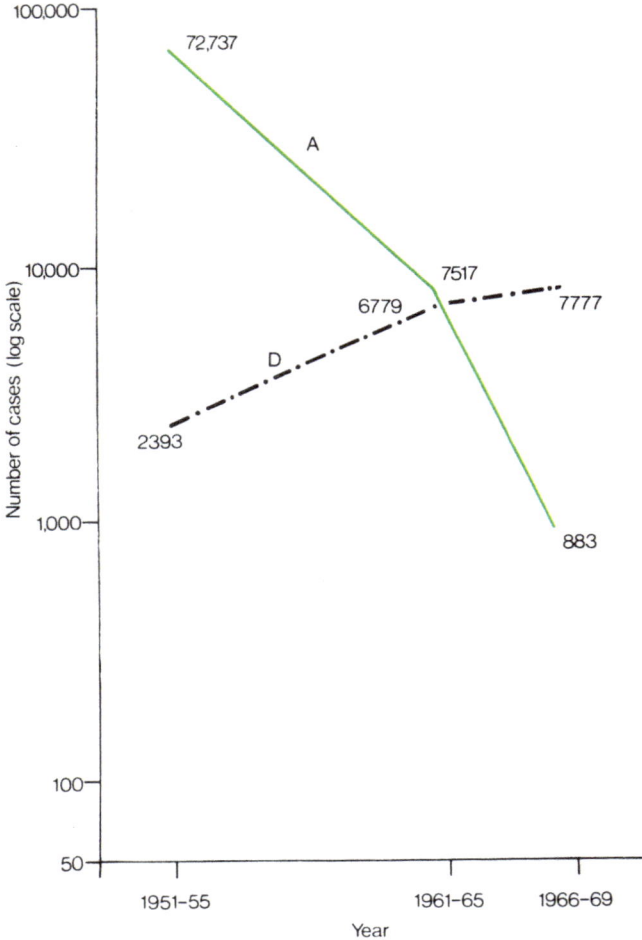

Figure 14. *Average annual number of poliomyelitis cases in 1951 to 1955, 1961 to 1965 and 1966 to 1969 in various groups of countries. A. 23 European countries, USA, Canada, Australia and New Zealand; D. 22 countries in Africa and 13 countries in Asia. (Data from* WHO.*)*

Contraindications

OPV should not be given to unhealthy people without careful consideration nor to anyone with acute or intercurrent illness, including diarrhoea or other intestinal dysfunction.

Paralysis following OPV is more common in antibody deficient patients than in the rest of the population. It should not be given to severe hypogammaglobulinaemia subjects, for they appear more liable to develop paralysis after exposure to both vaccine and 'wild' strains. Moreover, they may become prolonged high-titre carriers of virus in their gastrointestinal tracts.

It should not be given either to patients on corticosteroids or immunosuppressive therapy (who may best be immunised with IPV) or to pregnant women earlier than the fourth month.

The Future

More use might be made of dip/tet/pert/polio vaccine or of dip/tet/polio vaccine. Quadruple vaccine was extensively tested in Northern Ireland but was withdrawn because of problems of reactions to the pertussis component. A similar type of vaccine with an apparently acceptable pertussis compoent is in use in parts of Canada (Table 12) and the Netherlands.

Studies have also been made with dip/tet/pert/polio/measles vaccines and there is no reason why dip/tet/pert/polio/measles/rubella vaccines should not be developed for they do not require the rigid 'cold chain' in their transport, which is required for live virus vaccines, and could be of particular value in tropical countries as well as reducing the visits, in temperate climates, to immunisation clinics to three or four throughout childhood.

Most doctors now entering general practice may never see a case of paralytic poliomyelitis, but many of them were born in a year when 5,500 paralytic cases were notified in England and Wales alone, of whom more than 700 died. Truly, poliovaccine has been a success story, but the stability of the neurovirulence of OPV presents a continuous problem not found with IPV, and must be carefully monitored.

8. Measles

The development of measles vaccine followed rapidly on that of poliomyelitis vaccine. The techniques for manufacturing were similar, and the criteria for the acceptability of live virus vaccines, as far as safety and immunogenicity were concerned, had already been worked out from experience with poliovirus vaccines. Indeed, in some respects it has become easier to make virus vaccines than to know to whom they should be given.

Natural History

In developed countries, as exemplified by the UK and USA, the incidence of measles is highest in the three to five years age group in contrast to Nigeria where 50 per cent of children become infected by two years of age, and 75 per cent by three years. Unlike many infections, the disease is nearly always a clinical one, and before the introduction of vaccine nearly all children had had an attack of measles before puberty, and this provided a lifelong immunity to measles in almost all.

Notifications

Since 1940 when measles became notifiable in England and Wales the incidence has varied from year to year. There was an obvious biennial cycle but no evidence of any decrease in the total number of cases notified (which was more than 500,000 in alternative years) until immunisation was introduced in 1968. Before immunisation, because most people have an attack of measles in childhood, the total number of cases of measles in any country should be about the same as the number of births. It must be concluded that in many developed countries only about half of the cases are notified.

Deaths

Since the beginning of the century the number of deaths from measles in England and Wales has fallen from over 300 to less than one per million. This pattern has been similar in the USA. This decline in mortality started long before there were any effective drugs for the treatment of complications, and there is no clear evidence that the introduction of sulpha drugs or penicillin had any marked influence on the mortality. The prophylactic use of antibacterial drugs in a healthy child with measles may do more harm than good, and the routine use of antibacterial drugs is not recommended. However, it seems from studies done by the British Royal College of General Practitioners that antibiotics and sulphonamides may be of benefit to children who are sickly when infected with measles.

In the past, about half those who died of measles seemed to have had some other serious disability or chronic disease. The Registrar General's Decennial Supplement for 1931 for England and Wales showed that the mortality from measles of children aged one in social class V was about 20 times greater than those of the same age in social class I. Over the years better social conditions (including better medical care) have played the most important part in the reduction of measles mortality.

How Serious is Measles?

In developed countries measles seems to have become a relatively benign disease in recent years. Although exaggerations of the normal involvement of the respiratory tract are quite common, there is very little accurate information on the number of complications. A postal survey carried out in 1963 in England and Wales suggested that respiratory infections occurred in 38 cases, otitis media in 28 and 'neurological illness' in four per 1,000 cases. The exact definition of 'neurological illness' was unsatisfactory, although it was said that about 1 in 1,000 children with measles showed some impaired consciousness or evidence of encephalitis. Postal surveys of this sort have great limitations and the true incidence of neurological complications associated with measles infection is probably more in the region of 1 in 10,000 than 1 in 1,000 but varies with time and place.

When it was proposed to introduce routine measles vaccination in the UK, I questioned the advisability of this decision. Was measles vaccine required for healthy children? I felt that we should use it selectively for those children who might react severely to infection with measles, for children living in institutes and homes, and for any child who had reached primary school age without having had a clinical attack of measles, but this was a minority view.

Now that measles vaccine has been recommended for routine use we must encourage its use for all children who have not had a natural infection. Otherwise, as measles becomes controlled, they will grow up having had no contact with wild measles virus and a natural infection incurred as an adolescent or an adult may be more of a nuisance and more severe than an infection in childhood. Furthermore, it is said that the incidence of measles encephalitis in children over 10 years of age is 'considerably higher' than in younger children.

Vaccines
Live Measles Vaccine

The earliest attempts to vaccinate against measles were made by Dr Francis Home in Edinburgh in 1758 who tried to modify the disease by the inoculation of blood from a patient. (This method was presumably influenced by variolation.) However, it was not until the virus was adapted to grow in tissue cultures that the preparation of vaccine became practicable.

The earliest experimental vaccine was prepared from a strain of virus derived from a patient (called Edmonston) which became attenuated by being passed through human and chick-embryo tissue cultures. This attenuated strain produced about a 95 per cent antibody conversion rate but also produced fever, rash, upper respiratory symptoms and some-times convulsions in a high proportion of immunised children. The 'vaccine disease', although non-communicable, was too like the natural infection. Attempts were made to modify these vaccine reactions by giving an injection of pooled immunoglobulin at the same time as the vaccine, but this was hardly an acceptable procedure.

Attempts were also made to precede the injection of the attenuated virus vaccine by actively immunising with killed measles vaccine (q.v.) but this procedure produced some untoward results. Accordingly, attempts were made to develop further attenuated strains. The most satisfactory vaccine virus was developed from the Schwarz strain. This was a chick-embryo tissue culture (CETC) strain derived from the Edmonston B strain by repeated passages in CETC at low temperature. This vaccine produced fewer reactions but a seroconversion rate some-what lower than that of more virulent vaccine viruses.

Killed Measles Vaccine

Early experiments with killed measles vaccine (KMV) looked very hopeful. A course of three injections of formalin inactivated virus gave up to 95 per cent antibody conversion rates. Furthermore, there were none of the symptoms of mild infections with measles which followed the use of live attenuated strains. Unfortunately, when some children who had been immunised with KMV were challenged with live measles virus vaccine (LMV) they often developed what appeared to be an Arthus type of reaction (see page 29) with pain, erythema and induration at the site of inoculation. Some children exposed to natural infections developed very odd and sometimes severe respiratory conditions, urticaria and petechial and purpuric reactions. The reasons for this are uncertain but it would seem that after immunisation with the KMV available at that time, the original levels of neutralizing antibody fell rapidly but the individuals remained hypersensitive.

Another type of purified and inactivated vaccine was prepared from the haemagglutinin fraction of measles virus. Studies done with this type of measles vaccine included the trial of dip/tet/pert/polio/measles (see page 65) containing a haemagglutinin measles component. The seroconversion rates were good and no reactions occurred in the vaccinees when they were subsequently challenged with live virus, but the numbers tested were very small.

Routine Immunisation

The vaccine now recommended for routine use is a freeze-dried preparation which is provided with diluent and sterile disposable syringes. (The packages of vaccine and diluent should be stored in the cool part of a refrigerator, about +4° C. They should *not* be frozen as this is likely to crack the ampoule of diluent.) After the contents of the ampoule of diluent (Water for Injection) has been added, the vaccine should be used as soon as possible and certainly within one hour. The reconstituted vaccine may vary in colour from straw to pink.

Schedule of Immunisation

It is recommended that measles vaccine should be given in the second year of life (see Chapter 2). Due to the presence of maternally transmitted antibodies it often fails to immunise children under nine months of age. In many communities in the absence of epidemics it is advisable to postpone measles immunisation until about three years of age (because of fewer reactions in older children).

In areas where there is a high probability of infection at an early age, vaccine may be given as early as six months because of the variable seroconversion rate in children under one year of age.

In addition to routine immunisation in the second year of life, it is also important to ensure that all susceptible entrants to nursery and primary school are immunised: vaccine should be offered to any older children who have not had a clinical attack of measles.

Effectiveness

From field studies it appears that the overall protection rate[1] is in the region of 85 per cent. It seems reasonable to assume that protection will be durable, and fears of a waning immunity do not seem to be materializing.

With the present rate of immunisation there has been a considerable drop in the deaths from and incidence of measles. Unlike the achievements made with diphtheria and poliomyelitis vaccines, the eradication of measles seems a long way off. There is no use in hoping that when 75 per cent of the susceptible population has been immunised, measles, like diphtheria, will no longer be transmitted in the community. Measles epidemics have continued to occur in some communities with 75 per cent or higher rates of immunisation. However, such epidemics are separated by longer intervals and have tended to involve older age groups than before immunisation. In some places where immunisation programmes have been introduced measles seems to have become a low grade endemic infection.

It has been pointed out from a study of Bartlett's epidemiological model that in the UK there is a critical community size of the order of a quarter of a million above which measles can maintain itself more or less indefinitely in the population. In a population of that size there will be a sufficient number of susceptibles from those not infected in previous epidemics and from those migrating into or being born in the area. With populations less than a quarter of a million, measles could die out after an epidemic, and it would not recur unless reintroduced (as in the classical outbreak described by Dr Panum in 1846 in the Faroe Islands).

---

[1] Protection rates are calculated as:

$$\frac{\text{Attack rate in unvaccinated} - \text{Attack rate in vaccinated}}{\text{Attack rate in unvaccinated}} \times 100$$

After a partial vaccination programme with an 85 to 90 per cent effective vaccine, it has been predicted that the interval between measles epidemics will increase. Furthermore, relative to the size of the susceptible population, epidemics will be larger after vaccination than before (although smaller in absolute numbers). The previous biennial cycle may become a three to four year cycle and the age at attack will increase. As far as the critical community size is concerned this would increase as the immunisation rates increase. However, a vaccine acceptance rate of perhaps 100 per cent (with a 90 per cent effective vaccine) might be required to increase the critical community size above the total population in a homogeneous community. With the lack of homogeneity of the population a lower rate would presumably be adequate. Even so, the possibility of reintroduction will be present for years to come and to prevent outbreaks of measles after importations, a very high level of immunisation will have to be maintained.

'Fire Brigade' Action

In countries with well-developed immunisation programmes and good vaccine coverage it would seem sensible to invoke the 'fire brigade' technique. When cases occur in any district, immediate steps should be taken to immunise home, school, playmate and other community contacts. As with poliomyelitis control, the extent of the operation will depend on local conditions.

Reactions

The available vaccine produces a number of reactions. These are most marked in young infants and diminish up to three or four years of age which may be a more suitable age to offer vaccine in the UK.

Most children have some malaise, a transient rash and a mild febrile reaction about five to ten days after immunisation. The febrile reaction seldom lasts for more than 48 hours. More severe reactions—convulsions and encephalitis—have been reported in some cases. The onset of convulsions most frequently occurs between the sixth to the ninth day after immunisation. However, it is not easy to get accurate data on the number of these reactions, for convulsions may follow any inoculation by chance. Although general practitioners in England and Wales were asked to report severe and unusual reactions when the vaccine was introduced, the rate of convulsions in immunised children under two years of age reported was 19 per 100,000 which is one-tenth of the rate reported in the MRC trial of the same measles vaccine.

The occurrence of 'encephalitis' is probably in the order of less than one per 100,000 vaccinees. However, this is merely an estimate and there is no clear guidance for the diagnosis of 'encephalitis'. It might be assumed that the vaccine has prevented about 10 times more natural cases of encephalitis than it has caused.

Subacute Sclerosing Panencephalitis (SSPE)[1]

The risk of SSPE following vaccination with live virus measles vaccine appears to be about one-tenth of the risk associated with 'wild' measles virus. Indeed with the drop in the incidence of measles in countries with immunisation programmes, SSPE is apparently becoming even more rare than in the past. Measles vaccine significantly reduces the chance of developing SSPE.

Very rarely there have been reports of a nephrotic syndrome after measles vaccination. Any such cases should be discussed with an immunologist so that they can be immediately investigated.

Contraindications

Measles vaccine is contraindicated in children suffering from any acute illness. No adverse effect has been reported in egg-sensitive children because egg albumen and yolk are absent from the cultures. Careful consideration should be given to the immunisation of children with a history or a family history of convulsions or allergic disease. Vaccination should be delayed in such children until they are two or three years of age and it should be followed by an adequate course of an anticonvulsant, e.g. phenobarbitone for two weeks. This vaccine is absolutely contraindicated in children suffering from leukaemia, Hodgkin's disease, or other diseases of the lymphoid or mononuclear phagocytic system (reticuloendothelial system). Children with deficiencies of immune mechanisms or undergoing corticosteroid or immunosuppressive therapy should not be vaccinated.

Special Cases

Immunisation is particularly important in institutions for children who are malnourished (see Chapter 15) and for those with chronic diseases, e.g. heart disease and cystic fibrosis. Where immunisation is contraindicated adverse reactions can be reduced by the simultaneous injection of 0.6 mg per pound body-weight or 0.04 ml per kg body-weight of immunoglobulin in a separate syringe.

---

[1] SSPE is a latent infection of the brain with measles virus.

Since measles inhibits the response to tuberculin, tuberculin-positive individuals may become tuberculin-negative for up to a month after infection or immunisation with measles virus. Exacerbation of tuberculosis might occur with measles or measles vaccine, and therefore individuals known to have active tuberculosis should be under treatment when vaccinated. The value of measles vaccine far outweighs the theoretical hazard of potential exacerbation of unsuspected tuberculosis. Live measles vaccine given shortly after exposure to measles can provide protection and if a natural infection is prevented it should also produce durable protection.

While, as noted, live virus vaccines are not generally recommended for pregnant women, there is no evidence that measles vaccines may not be given safely and effectively to pregnant women who have been exposed to measles; however, on theoretical grounds it may be wiser to passively immunise with immune globulin susceptible pregnant women exposed to measles (see Chapter 14).

9. Rubella

Rubella is a relatively unimportant disease of late childhood and adolescence. It has often been said that rubella is not as infectious as measles but with the availability of diagnostic techniques this view may have to be modified. It now appears that the diagnosis of rubella based on clinical grounds alone is frequently incorrect. Since it has not appeared to be highly infectious by person-to-person contact and predictable epidemics like those of measles have not occurred, there has always been a varying proportion of susceptible adults in any population group.

If a susceptible pregnant woman is infected with rubella, the fetus is at risk of infection which may result in retardation of cell growth and necrosis. It is estimated from the National Congenital Rubella Surveillance Programme (NCRSP) that in the UK in non-epidemic years there are about 200 to 250 cases of congenitally acquired rubella. Prospective data from the Collaborative Perinatal Research Study (CPRS) in the USA indicate that about 30,000 children had congenitally acquired rubella as a consequence of the 1964–65 epidemic in that country. In that epidemic 3.6 per cent of the pregnant women in the CPRS had rubella, compared with an infection rate of 0.1 to 0.2 per cent in non-epidemic years.

Other relatively unimportant complications include transient polyarthritis and polyarthralgia in about 15 per cent of infected adults. Very rarely encephalitis or thrombocytopenic purpura has been reported.

Susceptibility
Women of Child Bearing Age

The susceptibility of women appears to be variable and is dependent on race, social class and community. In the UK and USA about 15 to 20 per cent of women of child bearing age appear to be susceptible to rubella.

However, in certain groups, e.g. student nurses, about 40 per cent may be susceptible and in some immigrants, e.g. from the West Indies and Africa, there appear to be more susceptibles than in residents of the UK and USA.

Studies show that about 90 per cent of women with no clinical history of rubella are nevertheless immune. In contrast about five per cent of women who think they have had rubella are devoid of antibodies. Because of the apparent relatively low infectivity of rubella it seems that only about one in 10 susceptible women exposed to the disease becomes infected, either clinically or subclinically.

The earlier in pregnancy the infection, the greater the chance of fetal damage. If all minor late defects and fetal deaths are included, the total risk of fetal damage after infection in the first 16 weeks of pregnancy is estimated at 30 to 40 per cent. The frequency is about 80 per cent in the first four weeks of pregnancy falling to 30 to 40 per cent, 20 per cent and 10 per cent in the second, third and fourth months respectively. The true incidence is almost impossible to determine but useful information of any major changes should become apparent from the NCRSP and the CPRS in the USA, which are still collecting data.

It would appear from epidemiological and other data that about 80 per cent of mothers are infected from their own children. However, from a recent NCRSP report, it appears that about 48 per cent of these congenitally abnormal live births were first born. The reason for this apparent discrepancy is that many infections during the first pregnancy had presumably led to pregnancies which had not gone to term. A great deal more information on the incidence of congenital rubella is required with regard to race and social class.

Immunity to rubella induced by natural infection or by vaccine is not absolute and reinfections may occur. However, reinfections do not seem to be associated with detectable viraemia which would put a fetus at risk. If there is a rash and arthritis, viraemia should be assumed with the possible attendant teratogenic effects. Repeated reinfections may be required to maintain immunity to rubella.

Control

There are three approaches to the problem of rubella-induced congenital abnormalities—abortion, immunisation or immunoglobulin (which will be discussed in Chapter 14).

In 1975 the 50 States and District of Columbia reported 854,853 legal abortions to CDC but there are no data on what proportion were in association with rubella infections. In England and Wales in 1971 and 1972 there were about 2,500 abortions on *ground four* (i.e., a substantial risk of the baby being born abnormal). Of these about 60 per cent were for maternal rubella: about 20 per cent were in contacts and about three per cent had received rubella vaccine. It is obvious that rubella causes a large fetal wastage and obviously much misery. At the same time it should be remembered that mere exposure to infection does not mean an abnormal fetus and the rate of exposed susceptibles who become infected is only about one in ten. Of all congenitally abnormal babies born each year in England and Wales (10,000) only about 100 to 200 on average are caused by rubella.

Relatively simple laboratory tests are available which can provide evidence of a recent or past clinical or subclinical infection with rubella. The virus laboratory should be consulted in all cases where the termination of pregnancy is being considered, except perhaps in obvious clinical cases.

Vaccines

Vaccines are issued as freeze-dried preparations and are reconstituted before use with distilled water which is supplied with the vaccine. It should be inoculated as soon as possible after reconstitution. Vaccine and diluent should be stored in the cool part of the refrigerator (about +4° C) but should not be frozen as the ampoule may crack. Rubella vaccine is given subcutaneously.

At present only live virus vaccines are available. The viruses in common use are the Cendehill and RA 27/3 strains. The Cendehill virus was derived from the urine of a case of acute rubella and is grown in rabbit-kidney tissue cultures. The RA 27/3 strain was isolated from a rubella infected conceptus and grown in human diploid cells (W1–38). Although these viruses have been recovered from the nasopharynx of vaccinated individuals, in only *one* of more than 1,000 cases studied could the possibility of transmission of virus from a vaccinee to a susceptible contact not be altogether excluded. Transmission of virus to susceptible close contacts thus appears to be such a remote possibility that it can be regarded as irrelevant.

The RA 27/3 vaccine appears to be more likely to induce an immune response which is qualitatively comparable to that following the natural disease than other vaccines. However, it seems to be more likely to produce reactions in young women. Antibody titres after vaccination are usually about four to eight times lower than those following natural infections. As in natural infections, reinfection can occur in vaccinated individuals. While there is no substantial evidence to suggest that the developing fetus is likely to be harmed as a result of maternal reinfection, all such reinfections have, with rare exceptions, been subclinical. However, the higher frequency of reinfections after vaccination than after natural infection presumably reflects the lower levels of antibody which follow immunisation.

Follow-up studies have indicated that antibody persists for at least six years following immunisation.

Vaccination of Children

In the USA immunisation of children of both sexes has been recommended in the hope of reducing the reservoir of infection and diminishing the risk of children transmitting rubella to pregnant women. However, it does not appear that this approach will attain the objective.

In the UK rubella vaccination is offered routinely to all girls between 11 and 14 years of age. This selective immunisation is an attempt to ensure that in the future all women of child bearing age will be immunised. There seems to be little hope of attempting to eradicate rubella by building up a high level of herd immunity by widespread immunisation, and it is hoped that the continuous passage of virus among male children will maintain the immunity of immunised girls.

Although more data are required on the exact numbers immunised, it appears that uptake of vaccine by the 11, 12 and 13 year olds has been less than would have been hoped—perhaps less than one-quarter of those in that age group. The effect of this programme of immunising 11 to 13 year olds will not be seen for some years and unless the acceptance of vaccine is greatly increased, it may not have the desired effect in measurably reducing fetal loss and damage.

Vaccination of Adults

Women of child bearing age must be informed that they must not become pregnant for two months following vaccination. It is not yet known whether rubella vaccine virus has teratogenic properties, but virus has certainly been recovered from the decidua of at least one pregnancy terminated at eight weeks in a woman immunised at three weeks. Advice on contraception must therefore be given at the time of giving rubella vaccine.

Until immunity has been built up in adults following childhood immunisation programmes it is important that vaccine is made available to all women of child bearing age. It is not recommended that all women should be offered vaccine routinely because many could be pregnant at the time of or within eight weeks of immunisation, and perhaps only 20 per cent will be susceptible.

It is important to ensure that vaccine is offered to nurses and nursery staff, particularly those in health centres, general practices, paediatric, antenatal and obstetric units and also to all female doctors and medical students, not only for their own protection but to minimize the chance of transmission of virus to pregnant women. Male doctors working in units dealing with pregnant women should also be immunised and vaccine should be offered to susceptible women teachers in schools and in teacher-training colleges.

Immunisation has been offered in association with family planning clinics and also to women in the early postpartum period who must be reminded that the usual period of infertility after pregnancy cannot be relied upon and that they must ensure that pregnancy is avoided for two months after receiving vaccine.

When vaccine has been offered to some of these groups some have insisted that they must first be tested for antibody and that only the seronegative should be immunised. For various reasons this has resulted in a number of susceptible women not being followed up and immunised. The only point of doing the blood test is to ascertain whether or not a pregnant woman has antibodies from a natural infection before she is immunised and before she has become pregnant, for if she has, no question of termination of pregnancy need be considered. It would seem administratively better to take a blood test, immunise the patient, store the test material if it cannot be tested at once, and if the patient does become pregnant within eight weeks test the sample. If necessary another blood sample may be taken after vaccination to ascertain whether any antibody which was demonstrated after vaccination was there as a result of infection before vaccination, or has been the result of infection with vaccine virus. In the latter case the fetus may have been at risk and termination can be considered.

Reactions

The administration of vaccine to girls may be followed by mild symptoms such as fever, rash, lymphadenopathy or occasionally a sore throat but such complications appear to be rare. The only really trouble-some adverse reactions reported have been arthralgia or arthritis with pain and stiffness in the fingers, cervical spine, knees and ankles. These are uncommon in children but have occurred in one-third of immunised seronegative adult women. It seems sensible to advise very active females, such as physical training instructresses and physiotherapists, to take things easy for about a fortnight after immunisation. Any adverse reaction to the vaccine should be reported.

Contraindications

An absolute contraindication is pregnancy. There is no contraindication of vaccinating a seropositive woman. Other contraindications are similar to those outlined under measles vaccine.

Inactivated Virus

Little progress with inactivated rubella virus vaccines has as yet been reported. The development of such vaccines is called for and it would solve the problems of testing women and ensuring that pregnancies did not occur in women who had been given vaccine. It could be given as a combined polyvalent vaccine with boosters as required.

Combined Vaccines

Combination of live rubella/measles/mumps, measles/rubella and rubella/mumps vaccines have been recently licensed in the USA and appear to be effective.

10. Tuberculosis

Although tuberculosis has shown a continuing decline since the earliest statistics were available, it still causes more deaths than any other notifiable disease.

In the UK the decline in deaths increased in the years after 1947 when streptomycin, para-aminosalicylic acid (PAS) and isoniazid (INH) came into general use (Figure 15). However, the annual rate of decline has

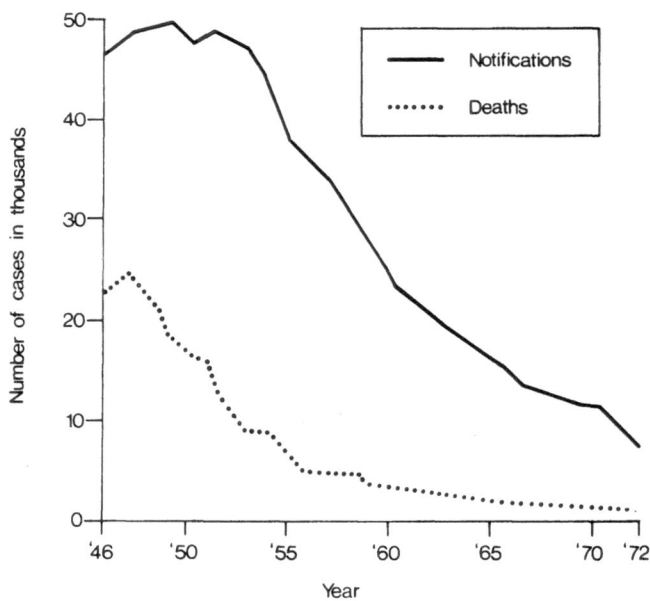

Figure 15. *Tuberculosis notifications and deaths, England and Wales.*

been markedly different in different age groups and in males and females. At present, deaths from tuberculosis in the UK occur essentially in males aged 45 years and over. In 1972, 92 per cent of deaths from all forms of tuberculosis and 94 per cent of deaths from respiratory tuberculosis (excluding late complications) were in that age group.

Notifications

Notifications (Figures 16 and 17) did not start to decline significantly until 1954, and even with improved ascertainment there was little decline in prevalence comparable to that of mortality.

Notifications are said to be a more reliable index of the present epidemiological situation of tuberculosis than mortality statistics. However notifications do not give a clear picture of the incidence of the disease because they indicate neither the onset nor the time of infection. The importance of notifying tuberculosis is that it helps to ensure immediate investigation of possible sources of infection. (Mass radiography findings offer another useful measure.)

In 1972 the national rates for all forms of tuberculosis were 22.8 per 100,000 population in England and Wales and 15.79 per 100,000 in the USA. These rates vary from area to area, reflecting urbanization and the socioeconomic conditions of several decades as well as of today. The reduction of tuberculosis has slowed down in some areas, apparently because of immigration. A recent survey in England demonstrated that 32 per cent of notified cases were in persons born outside the UK. The rate is said to be 27 and 54 times higher respectively for those born in India and Pakistan than for those born in England and Wales. Between 1965 and 1971 there was a decrease in notifications of about seven per cent per year among persons born in the UK but an increase of about 11 per cent per year among those born in Africa, India and Pakistan.

In a recent survey in the UK it was shown that about 20 per cent of all deaths from tuberculosis occurred in patients in whom tuberculosis infection was diagnosed *only* after death. Many of these deaths might have been prevented by better use of the facilities available for diagnosis and treatment.

Tuberculin Test

The tuberculin test plays an important part in the selection of individuals for immunisation with BCG (Bacillus Calmette Guérin). It is

Immunisation

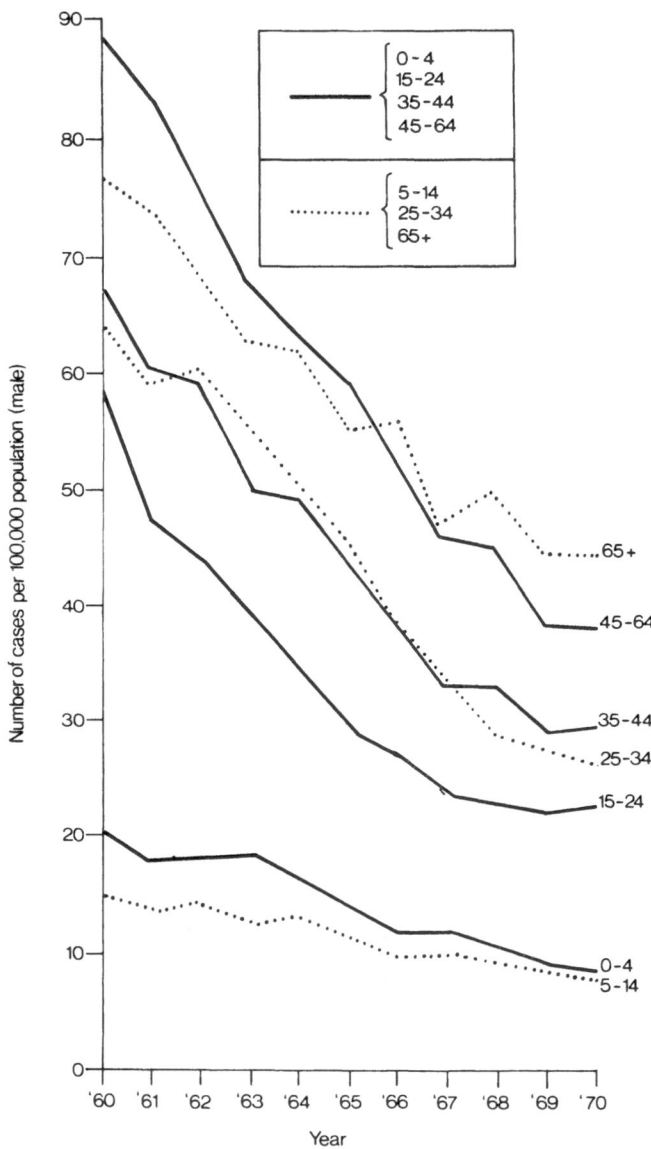

Figure 16. *Tuberculosis of the respiratory system: notification rates per 100,000 population in England and Wales (males). (Data from* DHSS.)

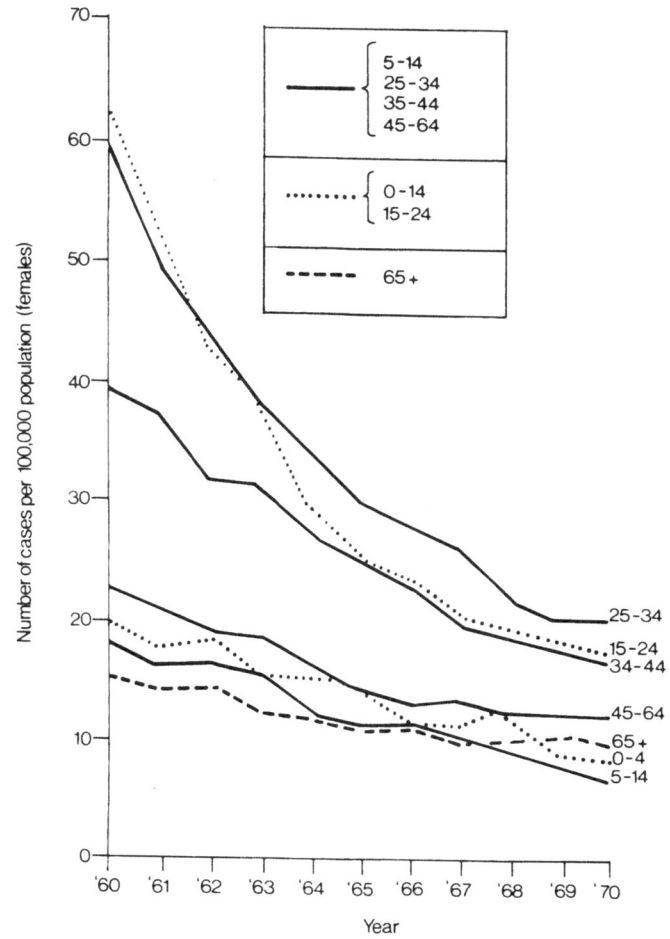

Figure 17. *Tuberculosis of the respiratory system; notification rates per 100,000 population, England and Wales (females). (Data from* DHSS.*)*

also used as a diagnostic test in individuals exposed to tuberculosis and for surveillance and epidemiological surveys. The test requires careful standardization and dosage because *most* people will respond if a sufficiently large amount of tuberculin is injected. Of the various types of tuberculin tests the intradermal (Mantoux) and multiple puncture (Heaf) are the most accurate and most commonly used. The test may be carried out with Old Tuberculin, but purified protein derivatives of tuberculin (PPD) are now commonly used.

Mantoux Test

In the Mantoux test a convenient dose is 10 TU[1] in 0.1 ml of buffer solution or saline injected intradermally with a very short (6 mm, 26 gauge) needle, usually into the left forearm, using a special disposable tuberculin syringe marked in 0.1 ml divisions.

Reactions

If the injection has been given properly a wheal of about 8 mm is raised which disappears within a couple of hours. Sometimes there is an immediate reaction of oedema and erythema which appears within 15 minutes of injection. This is followed by the characteristic delayed reaction which appears in most individuals with previous experience with mycobacteria. The time of its appearance and its extent give a measure of the degree of sensitivity of the individual. The reaction is usually at its maximum between 48 and 72 hours after the injection and consists of a central area of induration and erythema of variable diameter. In making a quantitative assessment of the test reaction, only the area of induration which can be felt and seen is measured. The reaction is usually graded as negative when there is no induration even if erythema is present. Only reactions with a diameter of 5 mm or more are acceptable as evidence of previous mycobacterial infection. A strongly positive reaction may be defined as 15 mm or more induration and should be referred for further investigation and supervision. A reaction of 20 mm or more is regarded as severe. Since it may be indicative of a tuberculous lesion somewhere in the body, individuals developing severe reactions should be given a thorough clinical and X-ray examination. If clear it should be repeated after six months. (It must be remembered that tuberculosis can infect areas other than the lungs.) A general reaction with fever accompanying a 15 mm or more Mantoux reaction is a strong indication of an active lesion somewhere in the body. If there is no reaction this indicates that the person has no tuberculous lesion in his body. However, individuals with immunological deficiencies or those suffering from serious illnesses may also have no reaction to tuberculin tests (see also Anergy, pages 73 and 86).

---

[1]One tuberculin unit (TU)=0.0002 mg of dried PPD.

Heaf Test

The Heaf test employs a simple and rapid technique in which a punch (the Heaf 'gun'), which has a ring of six solid needles, is released to a depth of 1 mm through a drop of full strength PPD or tuberculin containing 100,000 units per ml. (This must not be used for Mantoux tests unless diluted to 10 units/ml.) The drop should be placed on the arm with a sterilized glass rod or dropper.

Reactions

The reactions to the Heaf test are read in four to seven days (although positive results may appear earlier). If the result is negative, there is no induration nor are there any puncture marks or erythema. In a grade I response there are easily palpable discrete papules round some of the puncture points. With grade II there is coalescence of indurated papules to form a ring and in grade III there is a 5 to 10 mm wheal and induration. Grade IV is a greater reaction than grade III and shows a blister or central haemorrhage. A strongly positive reaction may be defined as grade III or IV and such reactors merit clinical and X-ray examination. As far as grade I responses are concerned, some consider that a Heaf grade I positive result at seven days is indicative of specific infection, and that in non-specific infections the response fades by three to four days. In deciding eligibility for BCG, Heaf grade I reactions are usually classified as tuberculin negative.

Tuberculin Sensitivity

It is now realized that low grade tuberculin sensitivity is partly tuberculous in origin and partly the result of natural infections with non-tuberculous strains of mycobacteria (including avian strains) and various atypical bacteria. Similarly, subclinical infections with atypical mycobacteria may result in enhanced resistance to subsequent infection with *M. tuberculosis*. Those showing a low grade reactivity to tuberculin (reacting to only 100 TU) have a lower incidence of tuberculosis in follow-up than do tuberculin-negative individuals. While there is a relationship between the degree of the reaction and the strength of the dose of tuberculin, of more practical importance is the fact that the degree of sensitivity gives some indication of the activity of an infection and the risk of subsequent complications and relapse. In England, children with a strongly positive result, i.e. an induration of 15 mm or more to 3 TU, were shown in an MRC trial to have had an annual rate of tuberculosis of 2.93 per 1000 during the first two-and-a-half years of the trial compared with 0.78 among those with 5 to 14 mm induration.

As indicated, notifications are not an accurate index of the incidence of the disease and this should be based on the results of tuberculin testing. The study of the numbers of tuberculin positive children from year to year in different ages and classes in schools has often given a valuable index of a source of infection to which a particular class has been exposed.

Control

Preventive measures depend on:

1. Detection of cases and their treatment.
2. The examination of contacts including tuberculin testing and chest radiology.
3. BCG vaccination.
4. Health education.

It would seem sensible to tuberculin test (and X-ray) all immigrants from countries with a high incidence of tuberculosis. Such a procedure could be compulsory on arrival to initiate treatment and prevent spread in the community. Although the disease may not become clinically manifest in immigrants until after a few years, identification on arrival could initiate immediate treatment and surveillance of contacts.

Anergy

Tuberculin 'anergy' (i.e. a non-reactor state) is present in the newborn and in the aged and in individuals with immunological abnormalities and tumours of the reticuloendothelial system. The tuberculin reaction also becomes negative after an attack of measles or after measles vaccination, and also in infectious mononucleosis. It is depressed in active leprosy and in sarcoidosis and in patients receiving steroid therapy.

Immunisation

Soon after tuberculin had been discovered and it had been demon-strated that tuberculous individuals showed increased sensitivity (Koch phenomenon), Robert Koch (1890) claimed that 'tuberculin' could be used for the treatment of early cases. However, this was soon discredited as was vaccination with other inactive preparations. It became clear that dead bacilli or extracts of mycobacteria would not stimulate immunity and that in order to be protected against tuberculosis it was necessary to have experienced an infection. This may be achieved by BCG or with the vole bacillus. These mycobacteria undergo a limited growth in human tissues and produce sensitivity and increased resistance to subsequent infection.

BCG

BCG was derived from a bovine strain of *Mycobacterium tuberculosis* by Calmette and Guérin. They observed that when bile was added to the medium in which the bacteria were grown, clumps of the microorganisms became dispersed and changes occurred in their morphology and virulence. They postulated in 1906 that prolonged subculture in such a bile-containing medium might produce an attenuated vaccine strain. After 231 subcultures over a period of 13 years the resulting strain was found to be harmless to man.

When BCG vaccine was introduced in the 1920s it was widely used in France where it was given orally. Although vaccination was popular, there were no statistically controlled trials and many considered the procedure unsafe. In 1930 BCG received a setback (as does practically every new vaccine) with the Lubeck disaster in which 73 infants (27 per cent) who had been fed the vaccine died. It was apparent that the children had accidentally been fed with a virulent strain of *M. tuberculosis* which had been kept in the same laboratory as the stock BCG strain. This disaster led to regulations controlling the production of BCG to ensure exclusion of all other strains and the WHO Expert Committee on Tuberculosis has repeatedly warned against the multiplication of laboratories preparing BCG vaccine. In the UK the vaccine is produced only by one commercial firm (Glaxo) and the entire production process is rigorously monitored. Many developed countries buy from reputable production centres elsewhere, and many developing countries obtain their supplies through UNICEF.

Inactivation of the liquid vaccine occurrs readily on exposure to light and to tropical temperatures. The development of freeze-dried vaccine, now in common use, which maintains its potency for at least 12 months if kept at $+4°$ C, has been of great importance in the efficacy of BCG in tropical countries.

Vole Bacillus Vaccine

The vole bacillus which is a murine type of *M. tuberculosis*, although of high pathogenicity for voles, was found to be relatively avirulent in common laboratory animals and man.

Administration of BCG (and Vole Bacillus Vaccine)

The vaccines are usually given by intradermal injection or by multiple puncture. The freeze-dried vaccine is reconstituted in saline and should be used immediately after reconstitution. The skin at the site of vaccination should be cleaned with ether or acetone but never with an antiseptic. 0.1 ml of the vaccine is injected into the skin just above the insertion of the deltoid, raising a wheal of about 8 mm. If BCG is administered too high, or too far forward or backward, the adjacent lymph glands (infraclavicular, cephalic, cervical or axillary) may become involved and tender. Complications seem to be more common if the injection is given into the skin of the thigh.

After about one week a red papule appears at the injection site. After three weeks a nodule progresses to a papule about 1 cm across or to a benign ulcer which heals in 6 to 12 weeks. No dressing should be used unless there is much discharge from the ulcer.

Vaccination of Babies

There is no point in doing a tuberculin test prior to BCG vaccination of babies because these tests are never positive in the first few weeks of life, even in babies of tuberculous mothers. With babies, great care must be taken to ensure that the inoculation is given intradermally and not subcutaneously which may give rise to a persistent local reaction. The dosage for small babies is 0.05 ml.

Multiple Puncture Vaccination

About a week after vaccination by multiple puncture technique, papules which are variable in number appear at the sites of puncture. They seldom show any obvious ulceration and heal with nearly invisible scars in about 10 weeks. This technique gives consistently good conversion which, although slightly less than that obtained by i.d. injections, is suitable for use by less skilled people.

Jet Injection

Provided jet injectors are properly maintained and continually monitored for consistent performance, jet injection could be a useful method for all age groups *except newborn babies*. It is generally painless and can be performed rapidly for large numbers by relatively unskilled personnel. The method has not, however, become generally acceptable because of the mechanical and maintenance problems of the apparatus.

Successful Vaccination

The success of the procedure may be judged by conversion to a moderate positive Mantoux reaction, three to four weeks after vaccination. This conversion is often slower in young babies, but it should occur in 100 per cent of those vaccinated with potent vaccine.

Abnormal Reactions

These may be local, regional or general. Untoward local reactions are perhaps most commonly caused by bad technique. There may be ulceration at the site of inoculation. This is best treated with a dry gauze dressing daily until the granulating surface is clean then application twice weekly of three per cent tetracycline ointment. Shallow ulcers with markedly undercut edges are slow to heal and healing is helped by application every other day of a solution of dimethyl sulphoxide to the raw surface and especially under the loose overhanging skin edge, followed by a compression dressing of gauze and bandage. This helps the loose skin to survive and stick to the underlying raw area. Once this has happened then application of three per cent tetracycline ointment will prevent gauze sticking to the remaining ulcer and healing will quickly follow.

'Lupus', eczema and keloid formation have occasionally been described. 'BCG lupus' is a persistent granuloma which always heals but often very slowly. Keloid is unusual in Europe but is said to occur with 'alarming' frequency in Israel. Some of the initial strains of the vole bacillus vaccine gave lupoid reactions but later strains appear to be free from that disadvantage.

An abscess may develop at the inoculation site, usually due to too large a dose or too deep an injection. These abscesses are usually sterile and heal rapidly once the necrotic material has been drained.

Lymphangitis and severe adenitis (with or without caseation) may follow a misplaced injection, but mild regional adenitis is so common following vaccination that it can be regarded as normal. In severe reactions showing streaks of lymphangitis there is sometimes a tendency to administer antibiotics or antihistamine. These are said not to help but the application of two per cent steroid ointment may be of value. Adenitis is less frequent after vaccination with the Heaf gun.

General untoward reactions are rare. About 15 fatalities following BCG, due to widespread dissemination of the organism, have been reported in the world literature: most if not all of them have occurred in individuals with immunological abnormalities.

Evaluation of Vaccines

There has been much controversy as to the efficacy of BCG and very discrepant results have been reported from different countries. Although some trial results have seriously questioned its efficacy, BCG has continued to be used extensively in many countries.

The existence of non-tuberculous mycobacterial infections in man and their immunological interaction with *M. tuberculosis* and BCG at the level of protective immunity and delayed-type hypersensitivity has helped to explain the apparent discrepancies in the tests of the effectiveness of BCG. Although the UK was about the last country to introduce immunisation as a routine measure, the best recorded trial of BCG and of the vole bacillus vaccine is being carried out in England. This trial has involved more than 50,000 schoolchildren and was started in 1950. After 15 years the protective efficacy appears to be about 80 per cent. This was similar in both sexes and extended to all forms of tuberculosis. It rose to a peak at two-and-a-half to five years after vaccination and then decreased. The data in the report indicated a low level of protection 12.5 to 15 years after vaccination. However, such an interpretation would be unwise because of the small numbers involved and because it is not reasonable to consider three years in isolation.

The efficacy of BCG vaccine in different parts of the world has varied from nil in a trial in Georgia schoolchildren (1947), to 31 per cent in Puerto Rican schoolchildren (1940 to 1951) and approximately 80 per cent protection in American Indians (1935 to 1938) (Table 13). It has been suggested that these differences are not only due to infections with atypical mycobacteria but are also due in part to differences in the potency of the vaccines used. (Atypical mycobacteria provide a partial natural immunity to which BCG can add little in populations with much atypical mycobacterial infection.)

Another intriguing possible explanation of the differences in the efficacy of BCG was proposed by Dr Ian Sutherland (see Table 13). He suggested that the efficacy of potent BCG is closely dependent on the extent of 'superinfection' of the vaccinated subjects and that the efficacy

Table 13. Rate of tuberculosis and protection afforded by BCG in various populations (from Sutherland 1971).

	Tuberculosis in unvaccinated (per 1,000 per year)	Protection from BCG (percentages)
N. American Indians	15.6	80
Chicago infants	2.2	75
British schoolchildren	1.3	78
S. Indian rural population	0.86	60
Puerto Rican children	0.43	31
Georgian (Alabama) population	0.13	14
Georgian schoolchildren	0.11	0

Data from Sutherland (1971), *Tubercle*, **53**, 110.

may fall off rapidly in the absence of boosting by virulent *M. tuberculosis* in the community.

It has been estimated that in England between 1970 and 1980 the annual incidence of tuberculosis in unvaccinated subjects will be between 0.04 and 0.1 per 1000. These estimates are just below the lowest figure (0.11) in Table 13. If Sutherland's hypothesis is correct, it might be expected that in future routine BCG vaccination in the UK will make virtually no contribution to the reduction of tuberculosis. However, before a firm conclusion can be reached, accurate data on the present risk of tuberculosis are required. It has been calculated that in the UK, routine use of BCG in 13 year olds in the 1970s would reduce the annual notification rate for negatives from about one to less than 0.2 per 10,000, i.e. vaccinating 10,000 children might prevent 10 cases in the next 10 years. By the 1980s, the reduction in notifications through using BCG is estimated at about 0.4 per 10,000 per year. This means that about four cases could be prevented in the following 10 years by vaccination of 10,000 13 year olds. By the late 1980s, the vaccination of 10,000 13 year olds would prevent only one case in the following 10 years. Obviously routine immunisation will soon be abandoned.

Who Should be Immunised?

In the UK, BCG is at present offered to tuberculin-negative children of 10 to 13 years of age but it would seem that this has a limited future as a routine measure for all children.

Selective Immunisation

BCG should be offered to those living in crowded conditions in urban communities, and to all immigrants and their children from countries with a high incidence of tuberculosis. They should be tuberculin tested before vaccination with the exception of newborn babies who should be vaccinated without delay.

All hospital workers who come into contact with patients, i.e. doctors, nurses, medical students, laboratory staff and necropsy attendants should be given a tuberculin test. In Europe it is usually recommended that all those who are tuberculin-negative or weakly positive should be given BCG. In the USA there is a strong body of opinion that such individuals should be kept under regular medical supervision and be periodically tuberculin tested: I subscribe to that view.

All persons going to work in developing countries of high prevalence of the disease should be offered vaccine if tuberculin-negative.

All contacts of known cases of tuberculosis should be vaccinated. With children it is customary to tuberculin test the child, and if negative to remove the child from contact where possible and then vaccinate following a second tuberculin test. The reason for the second test is to minimize the possibility that the child is naturally infected at the time of the tuberculin test. If the child was infected prior to the first test, the result might be negative because allergy had not developed. Babies should be similarly treated but without prior tuberculin testing. Tuberculin conversion may be detected by six weeks after vaccination, so ideally possible contacts should be segregated from exposure for that time. If segregation is not possible, and if isoniazid is to be given prophylactically, the use of isoniazid-resistant BCG should be considered.

High-risk group individuals who have been vaccinated in the past but have reverted to being tuberculin-negative may be revaccinated.

Contraindications

Positive reactors should not be vaccinated nor should children with a known immunological abnormality. Those suffering from any infectious disease, e.g. measles or whooping cough, or receiving corticosteroids or other immunosuppressive drugs should not be given BCG. As noted, weak positive reactions are no longer regarded as a contraindication to vaccination.

BCG has been given at the same time as other live and inactive vaccines, but in general it seems wiser to allow an interval of three weeks between the administration of two live vaccines.

General Measures

Although in decline, tuberculosis is still an important and common disease in the industrialized countries, where detection of cases and examination of contacts and chemoprophylaxis are more important for the future control of this disease than vaccination. The importance of BCG for developing countries is discussed in Chapter 15.

11. Influenza

One certain fact about influenza is that it is an epidemic virus disease involving the upper respiratory system. There are all grades of severity but it is probably the most abused clinical diagnosis and is applied to all sorts of upper respiratory infections, pyrexias of unknown origin and various alimentary upsets. Outbreaks of 'gastric flu', in summer or autumn, whatever they may be caused by, are not due to influenza virus. This does not mean that an outbreak of influenza cannot occur in the autumn and it may be the harbinger of a more widespread winter epidemic. It has a wide spectrum of signs and symptoms but classically it is characterized by an abrupt onset of fever, headache, aches in the limbs, and respiratory tract catarrh often with a hoarse cough.

Influenza is highly contagious and one should be very sceptical of diagnosing influenza in isolated cases or individual family outbreaks.

The annual number of days claimed for sickness benefit due to influenza in the UK in the past 20 years has varied from about 6 to 26 million. The United States National Health Survey estimated that with the advent of influenza A2 virus in 1957 during the eight weeks from 29 September to 23 November there were 70 million new cases with 'bed disability' and a peak of 12 million in the week of 13 October. Nearly 70,000 deaths were attributed to influenza in the USA in 1957 to 1958. As well as much morbidity, influenza also produces considerable mortality, particularly in the elderly and those suffering from chronic disease. In England and Wales in a fairly 'good' winter perhaps 3,000 to 4,000 old or debilitated individuals die of influenza.

History

In 1427 in the reign of Henry VI, an unknown chronicler in St Albans wrote 'Quaedam infirmatas reumigata invasit totum populum ... et sic senes cum junioribus inficiebat quod magnum numerum ad funus letale deducebat'. This states the essential features of an influenza epidemic and implies the sudden outbreak of a widespread infection with the highest mortality in the very old and the very young. This has been a feature of the mortality pattern of all recorded outbreaks except that of 1918 to 1919 when there was a high mortality in young adults which has never been satisfactorily explained (Figure 18). Epidemics of influenza appear to have occurred at various intervals from the 15th century to the 19th century. In 1840 following a number of years with no influenza, there was a pandemic of 'Russian flu', so-called because of its supposed place of origin. This was followed by pandemics of the 'Spanish flu' in 1918, which is estimated to have killed 20 million people, the 'Asian flu' of 1957 which circled the world within the year, and the 'Hong Kong flu' of 1968. In addition to these pandemics, epidemics and sporadic outbreaks have occurred at about one- to two-year intervals.

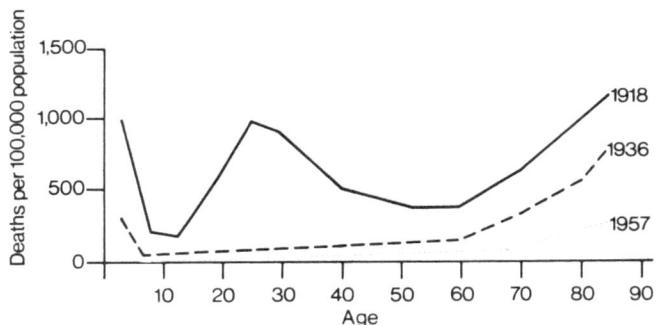

Figure 18. *Usual pattern of mortality from influenza in pandemic years compared with that of 1918. (Deaths per 100,000 population.)*

Influenza Viruses and Epidemics

There are three types of influenza virus: A, B and C; the latter appears to be of little or no importance. Influenza A virus is responsible for pandemics and for the widespread epidemics which occur every few years. They are reflected in 'excess mortality', i.e. when the number of deaths exceeds the norm for the given time and place. In contrast influenza B outbreaks spread less readily, are localized in nature and usually milder. They occur at about four-year intervals essentially in adolescents and young adults living in schools and institutes. Influenza B can occasionally produce large outbreaks and when such outbreaks are localized to closed communities the attack rates may be of the order of 50 to 60 per cent of the unprotected population.

Many virus infections, e.g. measles and mumps, are followed by a durable immunity because these viruses exist in only one immunological type. In contrast, not only are there two common types of influenza viruses, but there are various strains within each type. Influenza A viruses are very labile and major antigenic changes give rise to strains of which the world population has had no previous experience. Therefore, a recent past infection or immunisation with vaccines made from recently circulating viruses will not necessarily protect against new strains. The major changes in the virus which seem to occur about every decade are called antigenic 'shifts'. In contrast, minor changes which may occur about every year, called antigenic 'drifts', are sometimes so

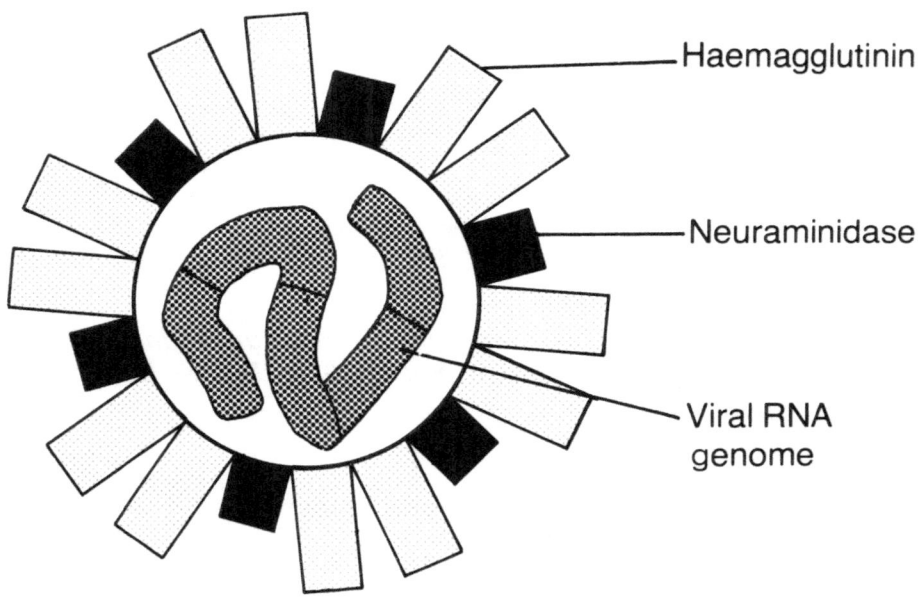

Figure 19. *Schematic representation of influenza virus.*

slight that a past infection with influenza or a dose of vaccine made from recent strains may protect. However, repeated 'drifts' may be summated over the years and markedly alter the antigenicity of any strain so that a vaccine made to an earlier version of the same strain may be relatively ineffective.

There are thus several possible reasons for the repeated outbreaks of influenza which occur in any community. There is more than one type of virus, and because of continual 'shifts' and 'drifts' the virus can find a population which has little or no immunity to the new strain even within a year of a previous outbreak. When an outbreak comes to an end as many as 60 to 70 per cent of the population may have had neither a clinical nor a subclinical attack, and there are thus plenty of susceptibles remaining in the population.

Structure of the Virus

Some clues to the natural history of influenza epidemics have come from studies of the structure of these viruses. They have a ribonucleic acid core which consists not of one single molecule, as in related myxoviruses, but of five discrete segments, and the great mutability of influenza viruses is presumably related to this. Surrounding the nucleoprotein is the viral envelope which contains two important antigens: haemagglutinin (HA) and neuraminidase (NA) (Figure 19).

Haemagglutinin

The HA haemagglutinates the red cells of some species in vitro because there happen to be specific complementary receptor sites on the red cells and on the virus particles. The ability to haemagglutinate forms the basis of an important test for studying the presence of antibody and for testing sera to determine the relationship of one influenza virus to another. If the antibody is specific to the particular virus, it will 'neutralize' the virus receptor and haemagglutination will not occur—so-called 'haemagglutination inhibition'. In vivo the haemagglutinin presumably plays a part in enabling virus to become absorbed and engulfed by cells lining the upper respiratory tract.

Neuraminidase

The NA may act on mucoproteins of the respiratory secretions and facilitate contact of virus and cell. More importantly, it may determine the amount of virus released by a given cell. Thus the higher the neuraminidase content of a virus the more readily it may be transmitted.

Changes in Virus Strains

Major changes in influenza A virus seem to be associated with major antigenic shifts in haemagglutinin or neuraminidase (Figure 20). When the various epidemic strains of recent years are examined it seems that the PR8 (Puerto Rico) virus which circulated in the 1930s could be described as A/H_0N_1. That type was prevalent until 1946 when FM_1

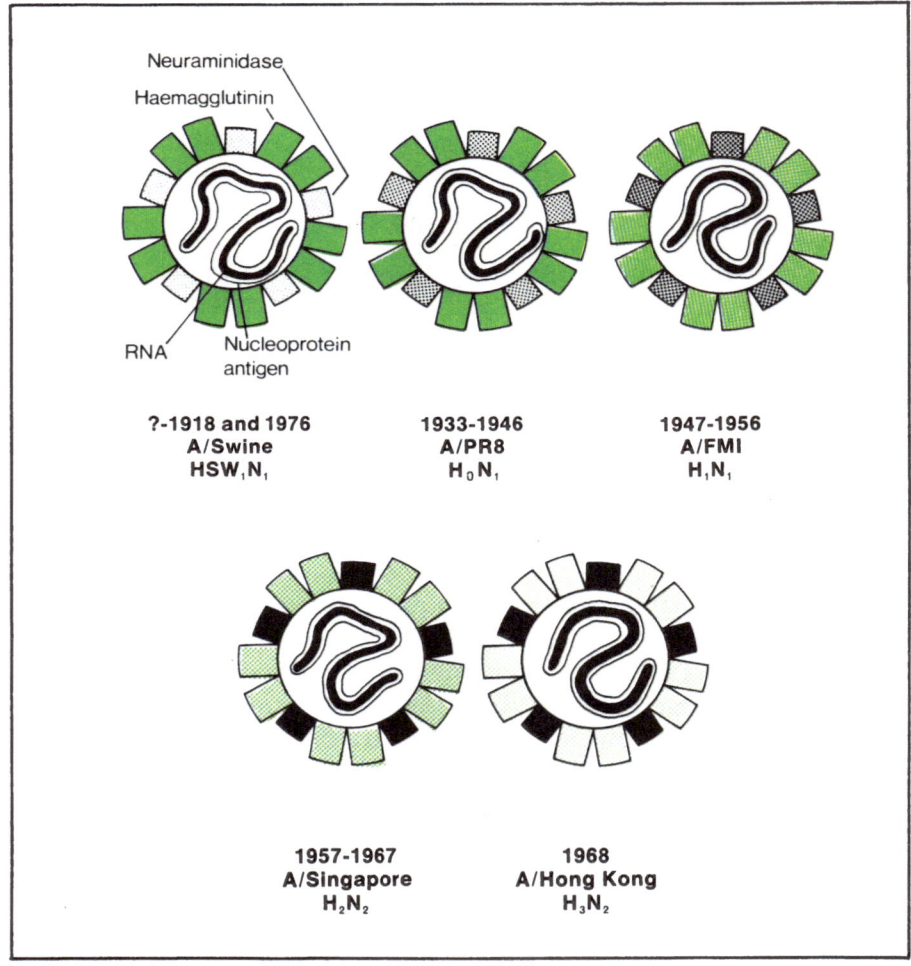

Figure 20. *A chronological representation of the changes in the surface antigens of influenza A virus since 1918. The nucleoprotein remains the same.*

(Fort Monmouth) type which is now identified as A/H_1N_1 appeared. That virus persisted with minor shifts in its antigenicity until 1957 when the 'Asian' flu caused by $A/Singapore/H_2N_2$ arrived. This was replaced by the Hong Kong virus H_3N_2 in 1968. It now appears that an H_1N_1 virus has turned up again. It is remarkable that when a new subtype of influenza A virus appears and spreads in man the old one disappears.

In 1976 a swine influenza virus HSW_1N_1 was recovered from military recruits at Fort Dix, USA. The virus is believed to be similar to the swine influenza of the 1918 to 1919 pandemic and appears to have been endemic in swine populations since 1918. This virus has not spread.

Influenza B viruses undergo occasional antigenic 'drifts' but not 'shifts' and in further contrast to influenza A virus several different variants of influenza B appear to circulate simultaneously.

Where do these new strains come from, and how do new subtypes spread in a community? Some people think that new subtypes represent recirculation of strains which circulated many years ago. As noted, H_1N_1 virus of 1946 and the virus HSW_1N_1 of 1918 seem to have reappeared. Similarly there is evidence that the Hong Kong variant was not a 'new' virus but had been circulating in 1890. No one knows the reservoir of the virus since 1890, but like the swine virus it could have been in an animal. There is some experimental evidence that some types of influenza A virus may be transmitted to swine, horses and other animals in which they may survive. Such viruses could return to the human population many years from now when the human herd immunity has fallen.

Another suggested explanation for the antigenic shifts is that they represent recombinant viruses consisting of a mixture (or hybrid) of an animal and a human strain. Recombination has been accomplished experimentally in animals such as swine and turkeys which had been inoculated with antigenically different viruses. The progeny of these different viruses had characteristics of each of the strains.

Antigenic shifts may be a survival mechanism of the virus. There are mutants in virus populations as in any other populations and when a particular strain passes through a human population and more and more people become immune only the mutants will survive in immune individuals. A population of mutant viruses will then gradually build up and give rise to a new strain. Why should this antibody 'drive' influence influenza and not other viruses? There is no evidence of viruses such as those of measles, mumps or rubella undergoing antigenic changes under the influence of antibody. Paradoxically, although influenza virus is a superficial type of infection with less contact with antibody-forming cells it seems to undergo mutational changes more readily.

It is difficult to assess accurately the duration of immunity to influenza virus because it seems to vary with different strains. The degree of immunity has to be measured by natural challenge and there is no suitable model in which to do this.

Prevention

With the exception of amantadine slow progress has been made in controlling the infectivity of influenza with antiviral drugs. Amantadine may be of some use in the prevention and treatment of influenza and has been recommended for high-risk patients who cannot or have not been immunised.

Theoretically, quarantine of infected individuals would control the source but this is not practicable with influenza. In a small island not dependent on world commerce all visitors could be excluded in the face of a pandemic wave of a highly lethal strain, but otherwise any other control of the human source is at present impossible. If it is discovered that certain animals are reservoirs of influenza virus some animal control might be initiated. As far as breaking the chain of infection is concerned in some countries, e.g. USSR, the wearing of face masks has been recommended during epidemics. This could interrupt the person-to-person spread of droplets, but an individual who had successfully protected himself from infection during work or travel might quite readily pick up virus at home from his family.

It is possible that in general children excrete larger quantities of viruses than adults and that they are the transmitters of infectious diseases par excellence. With influenza they may have had least experience with the viruses of the past and have no antibody to earlier related strains and little cell-mediated immunity. If this is so, it would seem sensible during outbreaks of influenza to try to reduce the contact between children and the elderly or the chronically sick. Influenza tends to have a higher mortality in the old and sick than in other susceptibles and 'flu (and other viruses) can precipitate an attack of bronchitis in those who suffer from that disease.

Immunity to Influenza

It would seem that antibodies to the haemagglutinin (HA) and neuraminidase (NA) play the most important part in protection. Anti-haemagglutinin antibodies have a greater antiviral effect than antineuraminidase. Since the HA and NA are constantly changing, the protective antibodies are of value for only a short time and absolute immunity may last only for about one year.

Evidence exists to suggest that an individual exposed to influenza virus will not only produce antibody to the infecting strain but will experience an anamnestic response of antibody to strains of the same group of viruses which had infected him in the past. The greatest response is to the most distant infection. This implies that influenza virus is an antigenic mosaic and suggests that the variations in HA and NA may be limited.

Although immunity to natural infection or experimental challenge is related to the possession of antibodies to the specific HA and NA of the challenge virus, presumably other factors are involved in protection, e.g. cell-mediated immunity.

Vaccines

The vaccines currently available in Western Europe and North America are inactivated virus preparations. The virus is grown in the allantoic cavity of developing chick embryos. The allantoic fluid is purified, concentrated and inactivated by formalin or some other inactivating agent. The haemagglutinin content is all important and the potency of the vaccine is recorded in haemagglutinating units.

Vaccine is given by deep subcutaneous or intramuscular injection (jet injectors have proved useful when large numbers are to be immunised but as noted require careful maintenance). Provided the current epidemic strains are included in the vaccine and there is good coverage of the exposed population, this type of influenza vaccine is claimed to have produced about a 60 to 70 per cent or sometimes greater protection. However, such protection is of limited duration, sometimes only about four to six months, although it may persist for up to five years following vaccination. One dose is usually adequate but if the anticipated epidemic strain is considerably different from recent strains, two injections at three to four week intervals are desirable. This will most certainly be required to produce protection against a new pandemic strain.

Reactions

Inactivated influenza vaccines sometimes produce redness and soreness at the site of injection, malaise, headache and fever. Children react particularly severely and doses for children should be smaller than the recommended adult dose. The reactions appear to be mainly due to non-viral protein although influenza virus is itself toxic. Some people used to say that 'the vaccine is worse than the disease'. While this may have been applicable to some vaccines in the past in a few individuals, considerable progress has been made to reduce reactions by purification using chemical techniques or zonal centrifugation.

In a recent mass vaccination campaign in the USA in which about 50 million doses of swine influenza vaccine were administered there was an increased incidence of Guillain–Barré syndrome. A case rate of about 1 in 120,000 adult vaccinees was observed, i.e. about 10 times that in non-vaccinated individuals in the USA.

Since the antigenic part of the vaccine is essentially the haemagglutinin, further efforts have been made to provide purified antigens by splitting the virus with ether or deoxycholate or by using subunit vaccines which contain only HA and NA. These are much less reactogenic than vaccines containing intact virus particles and should be more acceptable particularly for children.

To facilitate the administration of inactivated vaccines, and in the hope of stimulating nasal antibody (IgA), trials of giving the vaccine intranasally have been carried out. However, these have not shown any advantages in protection or antibody production.

Who Should Be Vaccinated

Although there was a nationwide immunisation campaign in the USA to vaccinate against the HS_1N_1 strain of virus, in Europe there seems to be no serious demand. When people are immunised because an epidemic is anticipated and it fails to materialize, they are less enthusiastic about being vaccinated the following year when an unexpected epidemic may occur.

The serious nature of influenza does not seem to be generally appreciated—one death from polio is headlined, a thousand from influenza go unheeded. Most people in Europe seem to be prepared to take the chance of not getting 'flu during the winter and do not bother about vaccine. Yet in an epidemic year, as in 1969/70, in addition to the increased mortality, influenza caused the loss of 25 million working days in England and Wales. Of some interest in this respect was one controlled study which showed that vaccination had saved about 14 working days per 100 employees. However, after the 'flu outbreak those in the placebo group who had not been sick during the outbreak had the equivalent time off 'sick'—but not from influenza!

It is difficult to evaluate the vaccines presently available in the general population, and there has been little effort to use them on a wide scale until recently in the USA with HSW_1N_1 virus. Following the recovery of this swine influenza a nationwide immunisation programme was put into operation. However, as already noted, the predicted spread of this strain in man has not occurred at the time of writing as it did in 1918/19.

In general there are problems involved in making enough vaccine, testing it and of its cost. It has been estimated that if the 'flu vaccines available were widely used in the UK it would probably cost about 30 to 40 million pounds per year not allowing for payments to general practitioners.

The vaccines available at present are not recommended for routine use in an attempt to control epidemics but are of value for 'high-risk' groups who should be vaccinated annually. They include:

1. Patients with chronic pulmonary disease, e.g. bronchitis (who are especially vulnerable to influenza and in whom influenza can initiate an exacerbation). Also, those with emphysema, bronchiectasis, pulmonary tuberculosis, cystic fibrosis, chronic asthma, and cardiovascular disease, especially those with mitral stenosis and with frank or incipient failure. Also included are patients with chronic diseases of the renal or nervous systems or with metabolic disorders.

2. Elderly persons particularly those living in institutions.

3. Children living in institutions, including schools, where high attack rates can occur because of the facility of spread.

4. Individuals such as doctors, nurses, ambulance men and other medical personnel who are at special risk of infection and workers in other 'key' occupations.

There is some controversy about immunising pregnant women and some experts do not consider this acceptable. There are conflicting reports on the possible incidence of congenital defects due to influenza virus but it does seem that in epidemic years there may be an excess infant mortality. If a pregnant woman can be prevented from having influenza this outweighs any upset which might be caused by the injection of an inactivated virus vaccine.

Contraindications

Vaccine should be used with caution in children because of the severity of reactions. They should be given appropriately smaller doses as indicated in the manufacturer's literature. The vaccine is contraindicated in individuals sensitive to egg products, poultry or feathers.

The disadvantages of the inactivated influenza vaccines at present available are the short-term immunity they produce since they have to contain the current strain, and the fact that their composition has to be constantly changed.

In spite of the problems, vaccines with a reasonable rate of protection for at least one season are available. These could be life-saving in the special groups mentioned above, and could allow others to maintain essential services in the face of an epidemic.

Future Developments

One of the problems in preparing vaccines has been the adaptation of a new strain to growth in eggs which delays production. It is now possible to combine current strains with an old well-established high-growth laboratory strain and to produce a high-yield virus with the antigenic properties of the new strain. This can make vaccine production with a new strain possible in a few weeks, rather than months, of adaptation of a new strain to produce a sufficient titre of virus. This recombination technique has made it possible to prepare viruses with the neuraminidase of one strain and the haemagglutinin of another and it is possible to swop virulence and other properties. It has been proposed that a 'library' of influenza viruses could be prepared which might contain the expected virus of the next epidemic. As soon as a new epidemic strain had been spotted and identified by one of the laboratories of the WHO surveillance network, a vaccine could be immediately manufactured.

With only a limited number of antigens—which seems a reasonable hypothesis because nature seldom has an infinite number of species or subspecies in any genus—it might be possible to make a vaccine containing all possible antigens.

Live Virus Vaccines

Live virus influenza vaccines have been most intensely tested in the USSR but the methods of controlling many of the studies have been unsatisfactory. Massive immunisation by aerosol vaccines in some cities in the USSR and also in Yugoslavia does not seem to have influenced epidemics to any great extent. Reactions in children to live influenza virus vaccines were considerably greater than in adults but vaccination by the intranasal route was said to have reduced these. The main problem was to attenuate the virus so that it would infect and immunise but not produce any disease. Over-attenuated strains which have produced no illness have not stimulated an adequate antibody response.

Theoretically, a live virus vaccine could be prepared in the face of an epidemic by mating the new virus with an avirulent well-adapted laboratory strain to produce an avirulent hybrid with the new antigens. A few thousand eggs could rapidly provide enough vaccine for millions of people and prevent many deaths in the face of a virulent epidemic. However, there are problems of safety testing and of transient immunity, etc. and the additional problem of the stability of such a virus when it replicates in man. Its potential for spread and mutation to virulence are unknown properties.

12. Vaccination for Travel

'Come to Carnival in Rio'
'Visit Sunny North Africa'
'Tour the Game Parks of Kenya'
'See the Taj Mahal by moonlight'
'And come home sick'
(B. G. Maegraith)

It is the duty of individuals travelling abroad to be aware of the measures they should take to protect themselves against the diseases prevalent in the countries to be visited or passed through. Their attention should be drawn to government pamphlets such as those provided by the US Department of Health, Education and Welfare or *Notice to Travellers*, obtainable from Health Departments in the UK. These give information on the distribution of most tropical and subtropical diseases and guidance on personal protection and on immunisation against them.

Because of changes in immunisation requirements, intending travellers to countries outside Europe and North America should seek information from the embassy or mission of the countries to be visited.

Diseases Requiring International Certificates

The health regulations of some countries require international certificates against smallpox, yellow fever and cholera from some travellers entering these countries. Some countries do not require vaccination certificates in the case of infants. If vaccination is contraindicated on medical grounds, most countries are prepared to accept a doctor's certificate indicating the reasons for not vaccinating the traveller (see contraindications). These certificates should be authenticated by the local authority as for WHO certificates. (There are three places—Libya, Australia and Singapore—which at present may not accept a doctor's certificate and this should be checked.)

Smallpox

Anyone travelling to an endemic country and also to many non-endemic countries still requires evidence of vaccination against smallpox.

Apart from a few cases of variola minor in some Somali nomads it appears that by late 1978 global eradication of smallpox will have been achieved. South America and West Africa have been certified free for several years, no cases have been reported from Asia since the end of 1975, and certification of eradication, i.e. two years after the onset of the last known case, has now been given there.

Strictly speaking vaccination should now be required only for travel in the remaining endemic area of Africa. However, some countries which have been free of smallpox for many years still require an international certificate from all travellers (except infants in some places). Others require a certificate from travellers who have arrived from an infected area. The countries requiring vaccination are changing and information on those which still require vaccination on direct flights from the UK and USA (or any other country) should be obtained from the relevant embassy.

Where there is a contraindication to vaccination a certificate by the practitioner on headed notepaper stamped by the local health authority is usually accepted at the port of entry. Contraindications etc. are discussed in Chapter 6.

Cholera

It would seem that until the beginning of the last century cholera was confined to the continent of Asia and was not a serious pandemic disease. However, in 1817 an extensive outbreak in the Ganges delta spread during the next six years throughout large parts of Asia and Africa and then disappeared. Following this, other waves of infection have spread from India and in the second and third pandemic, in the 19th century, the disease reached Britain. Canada and New York were infected by Irish immigrants fleeing from their native country. In the London outbreak in 1848/49 John Snow (of Broad Street pump fame) was able to show conclusively by applying the scientific method to the study of an epidemic that cholera was transmissible by faecal contamination of water. The causative organism *Vibrio cholerae* was subsequently identified by Robert Koch in 1881.

With the development of sewage disposal and water filtration techniques the disease tended to disappear from many countries and for many years the vibrio appears to have been confined to the edges of the Ganges and Brahmaputra rivers. Then in 1961 the seventh pandemic appeared. This was due to a new biotype called El Tor (after a quarantine station in Egypt). The pandemic started in Sulawesi in the

Indonesian Archipelago, spread throughout South East Asia in 1963, to the India–Pakistan subcontinent in 1964, the Middle East in 1965/66 and to Eastern Europe, West and North Africa and to Spain (Figure 21), threatening much of the rest of Europe and the Americas.

The El Tor vibrio, like other types, spreads from person to person and by contamination of water supplies and food leading to more explosive outbreaks. Nobody knows why the recent pandemic is so widespread but it seems that there are many carriers or symptomless excretors and many more mild cases of diarrhoea than occurred with the classical vibrio.

The extent of any outbreak following an importation will be governed by the standards of public and personal hygiene. All physicians must be vigilant about the possibility of importation by tourists and migratory workers, and cholera must be suspected in individuals with diarrhoea returning from an infected area. With the extensive movement of people nowadays, it has even been suggested that in a few years *V. cholerae* might be as common as *Shigella sonnei* in schools and institutes in Western European countries. Hopefully, as in other pandemics of cholera, it will disappear.

Prevention

Control depends on maintaining levels of personal and community hygiene which will prevent faecal–oral spread of the vibrios. Vegetables which have been irrigated with sewage, or shellfish from sewage-infected water, are potent sources of infection. In many parts of the world it is wise to avoid drinking unsterilized water, eating from street stalls, or eating green salads or fruits which cannot be peeled or have not been immersed in water-sterilizing solution.

Immunisation

Obviously in non-endemic countries there is no place for routine cholera immunisation and the only indications for cholera vaccine are travel to and residence in countries with the disease. Vaccine should not be used in managing contacts of imported cases or controlling the spread of infection.

Vaccine

The vaccine at present available is very similar to that introduced by Kelle at the end of the last century. It consists of phenol or formalin killed serotypes of *V. cholera* of the classic Ogawa and Inaba strains. (Vaccine prepared from the biotype El Tor protects against the classical

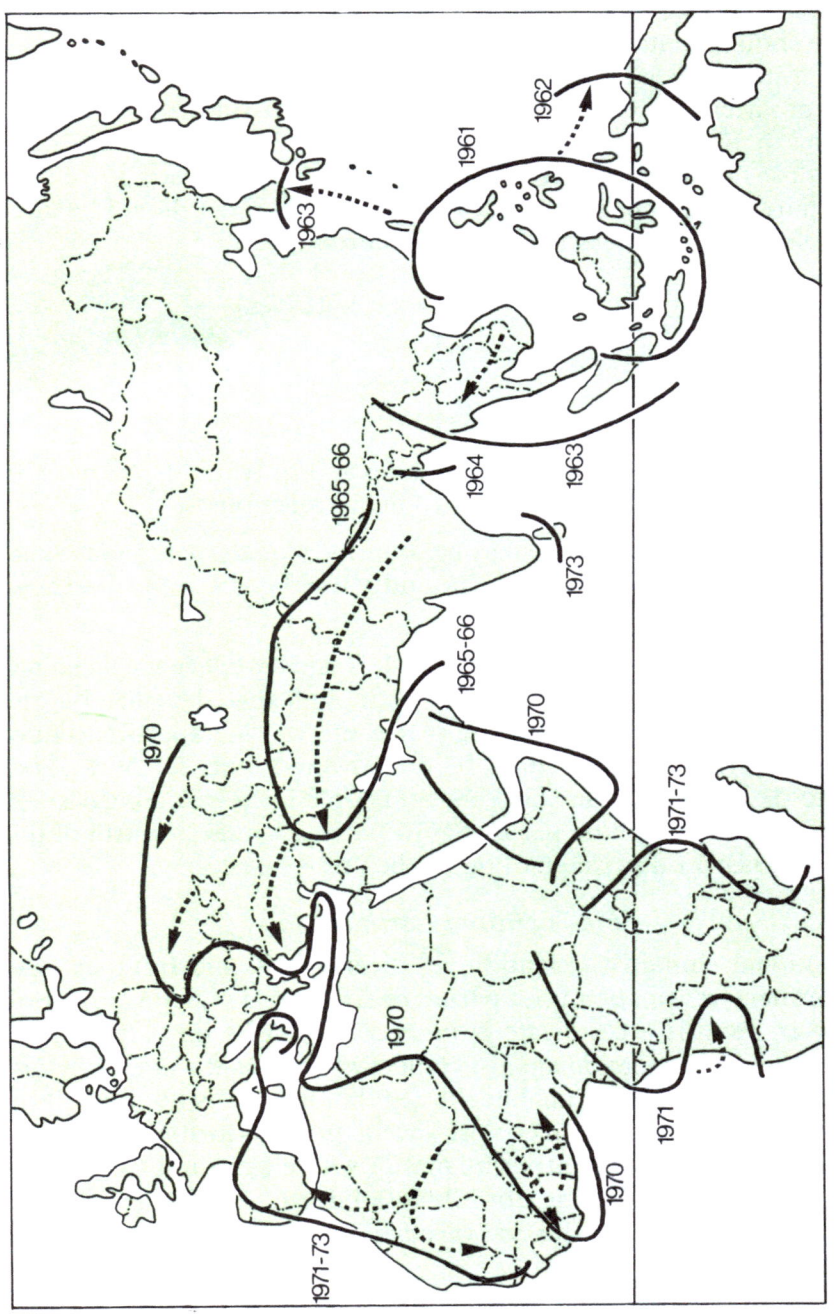

Figure 21. *Global spread of cholera 1961 to 1973* (WHO).

serotypes and vice versa.) The WHO recommends that each dose of vaccine should contain $4,000 \times 10^6$ organisms of each serotype per ml.

The usual dose is a subcutaneous injection of 0.5 ml followed by 1.0 ml of vaccine about three or four weeks later. In order to reduce reactions it may be given intradermally (i.d.), when the 0.5 ml and 1.0 ml doses may be replaced by 0.1 ml and 0.2 ml. Booster injections are required at about six-month intervals; 0.2 ml (i.d.) should be adequate. Suitable s.c. doses (in ml) for children are:

dose	<5 years	5–10 years
1	0.1	0.3
2	0.3	0.5
booster	0.1	0.3

The vaccine may be combined with tetanus and/or typhoid vaccine. The intradermal route is recommended to avoid reactions.

Reactions. Occasionally there may be some local tenderness and redness at the injection site. Fever, headache and general malaise and diarrhoea may occur.

Efficacy. The vaccine is of limited value. It is said to reduce the incidence of overt disease by 40 to 80 per cent, but this depends on the epidemiological situation: in some places the vaccine appears to have produced very little protection. Its effectiveness lasts for only about three to six months. It may not prevent people from becoming carriers and appears to be of little use in controlling epidemics. Control of this disease is based on permanent public health measures.

International Certificates

International cholera vaccination certificates are valid from six days after primary vaccination for a period of six months. On revaccination within six months a certificate is immediately valid for a further six months. Since vaccination against cholera is of limited value, a change was made in the international health regulations, and with effect from May 1973, it was agreed that cholera vaccination was no longer required for admission to most countries no matter where travellers came from. However, travellers arriving from cholera-infected areas may still have to provide evidence of cholera vaccination in Malawi, Papua, New Guinea and the Seychelles.

For travellers using the usual tourist accommodation the risk of cholera is very small. Otherwise, travellers to the Middle and Far East should be immunised for their own protection. They should have an international certificate to avoid any inconvenience.

Cholera sometimes reappears in countries which have been free of the disease for several years. As previously noted, when travelling abroad it is, therefore, wise to check with the relevant embassy regarding vaccine requirements. (Most countries require only one injection of cholera vaccine but some, e.g. Saudi Arabia, may require two.)

Yellow Fever

This is a disease with a haemorrhagic diathesis which gives rise to fever, haematemesis (the dreaded 'black vomit') and jaundice. The case fatality rate is from 10 to 30 per cent. In the endemic areas in Central and South America and in Africa between 25°N and 5°S (including the Sudan, Ethiopia and countries of West, Central and East Africa) (Figure 22) there is often a high attack rate with many subclinical cases in the indigenous population.

Epidemiology

At one time yellow fever was the scourge of West Africa (the 'white man's grave') and of the Caribbean. During the summer, the disease would spread from these areas by sea routes to coastal towns of Europe and up the coast and along the navigable rivers of North America. At the beginning of this century Walter Reed and his colleagues working in Cuba discovered that the disease was transmitted by the black and white stegomyia *Aëdes aegypti*. By controlling the breeding places of this highly domestic mosquito, General Gorgas eradicated yellow fever from the Caribbean in a few weeks and it was soon controlled in adjacent areas. However, the battle was not won. Although urban yellow fever is transmitted from man to man by *A. aegypti*, the reservoir of the virus is among monkeys of the central rain forests of South America and Central Africa where the disease is transmitted from monkeys to man by mosquitoes. It is obviously impossible to control the monkey reservoir or the forest mosquitoes, and the disease is prevented in man by immunising people living or working in the forests or on their edges, and visitors to endemic zones. (The virus from the forest can reach urban centres in the blood of infected people, and can then spread if there is inadequate control of *A. aegypti*.)

In recent years the virus has reappeared in southern Sudan (1940 and 1950), Panama (1949 and 1956), Ethiopia (1960–61), Peru (1969/70), Bolivia (1972) and Brazil (1973). In the Ethiopian epidemic there were

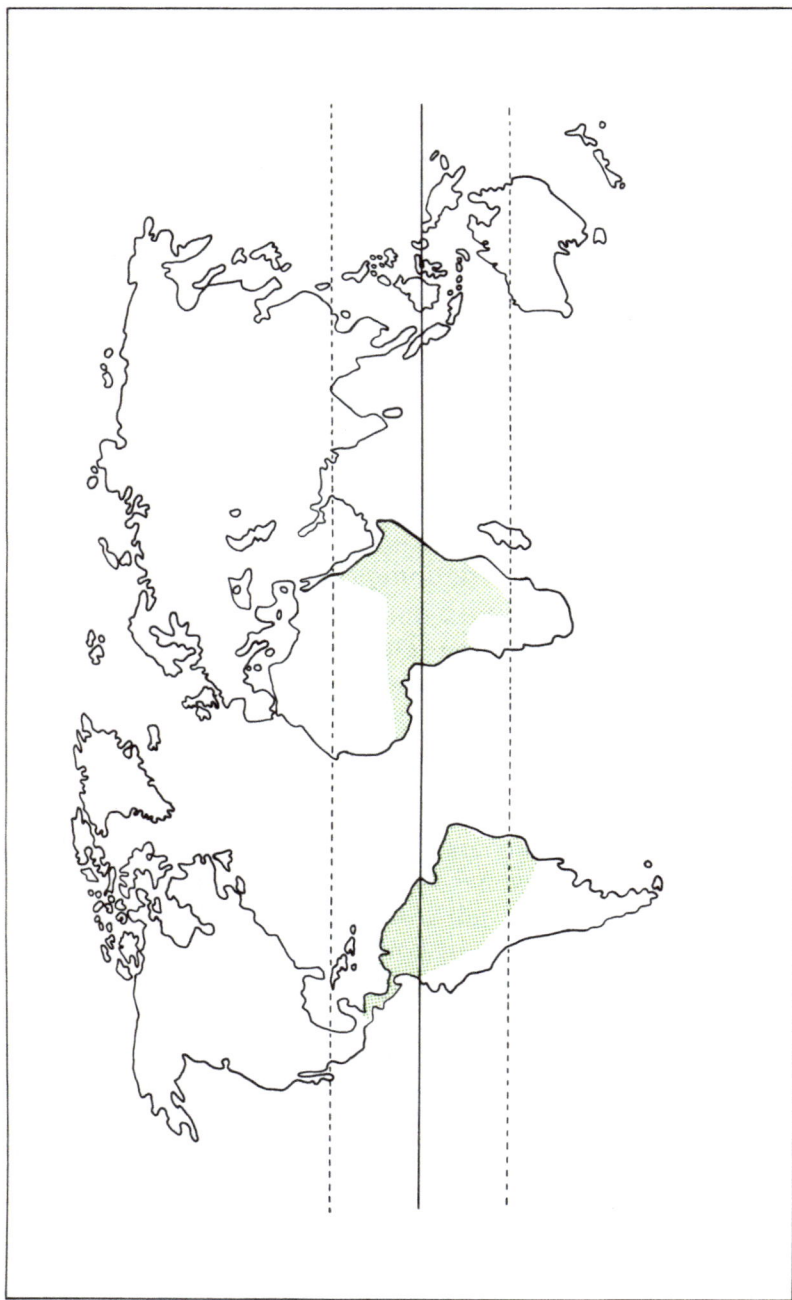

Figure 22. *Geographical distribution of endemic cases of yellow fever.*

probably more than 30,000 deaths. These and recent outbreaks in Senegal and in remoter parts of Nigeria, Ghana and the United Republic of Cameroon and Upper Volta, presumably represent a relaxation in immunisation programmes.

Yellow Fever Vaccine

Yellow fever vaccine consists of an attenuated virus (17D) developed by Max Theiler who repeatedly passed the virulent Asibi strain (recovered in West Africa from a patient of that name) intracerebrally in mice. The virus was further attenuated by passage in chick-embryo tissue culture. When this virus was injected into man, it replicated and circulated in the blood but produced no disease. For vaccine production on a large scale, the 17D virus is grown in the developing chick embryo. Earlier batches of vaccine were most probably contaminated with avian leucosis virus, but the 17D strain is now propagated in eggs from leucosis-free flocks. Human serum is no longer added as a stabilizing agent, for in 1942 it led to an extensive outbreak amongst American troops in Northern Ireland of jaundice due to contamination by hepatitis B virus. In this outbreak about 28,600 cases of jaundice occurred among 2.5 million vaccinated American troops, of whom 62 died.

The 17D vaccine used today is available only at designated centres. It is a freeze-dried preparation which is reconstituted in distilled water immediately before use. The dose is 0.5 ml and the vaccine may give lifelong immunity.

Contraindications

Unless specifically requested 17D vaccine should not be given to children under nine months of age since it may give rise to encephalitis in young babies. Vaccine should not be given to individuals who are sensitive to eggs.

Reactions

If the contraindications are observed, reactions are extremely rare. Very occasionally there may be a very mild local reaction at the site of injection or slight malaise about the seventh day after immunisation. (The 'Dakar' vaccine, derived from mouse-brain virus, is not recommended for elective use because it has produced encephalitis in vaccinated subjects and is considered too virulent.)

International Certificates

These certificates are available after vaccination at the relevant centre.

Immunisation

They are valid 10 days after primary vaccination and for 10 years thereafter, and immediately valid for a further 10 years on revaccination. Certificates are required for travel to or through the endemic zones, but not for Asia or the Far East *unless* the traveller is entering from a yellow fever area.

Simultaneous Immunisation

As already noted, in order to sort out any reactions it is best to allow an interval of three weeks between the administration of two live vaccines. However, if yellow fever and smallpox are required for immediate travel, they may be given at the same time in opposite arms. There is no evidence that if the interval is longer it will materially influence the antibody response.

Some interference between cholera and yellow fever immunisation may occur but it is not sufficient to influence schedules of immunisation, and yellow fever and cholera vaccines may be given at the same time or at any convenient interval.

When many immunisations are required, it is important to remember the time after immunisation when the validity of an international certificate begins, to arrange suitable spacing of the vaccines.

If the traveller is going to a smallpox endemic area, smallpox vaccine should be given first so that it can be repeated if it does not 'take'.

Typhoid Fever

Typhoid fever often presents as a pyrexia of unknown origin with a cough. It should always be suspected in a person with a PUO of three or more days who has recently returned from a holiday in an endemic area, e.g. the Mediterranean basin. Early notification of the disease should be made to the local health authority. This is particularly important when the holidaymaker has been on a 'package tour'.

The causative agents, *Salmonella typhi* and *Salmonella paratyphi*, are primarily human pathogens, unlike the more than 1,000 other species of salmonella which infect animals and cause food poisoning in man. Person-to-person spread of *S. typhi* is relatively unimportant, and outbreaks usually result from contaminated food or drink. Typhoid is predominantly a disease of countries where water supplies are liable to faecal contamination. Infected water may lead to outbreaks from contaminated milk, shellfish, corned beef, etc.

Epidemics of typhoid are rare in Northern Europe (Figure 23) and in North America but some readers will recall the outbreaks in Croydon

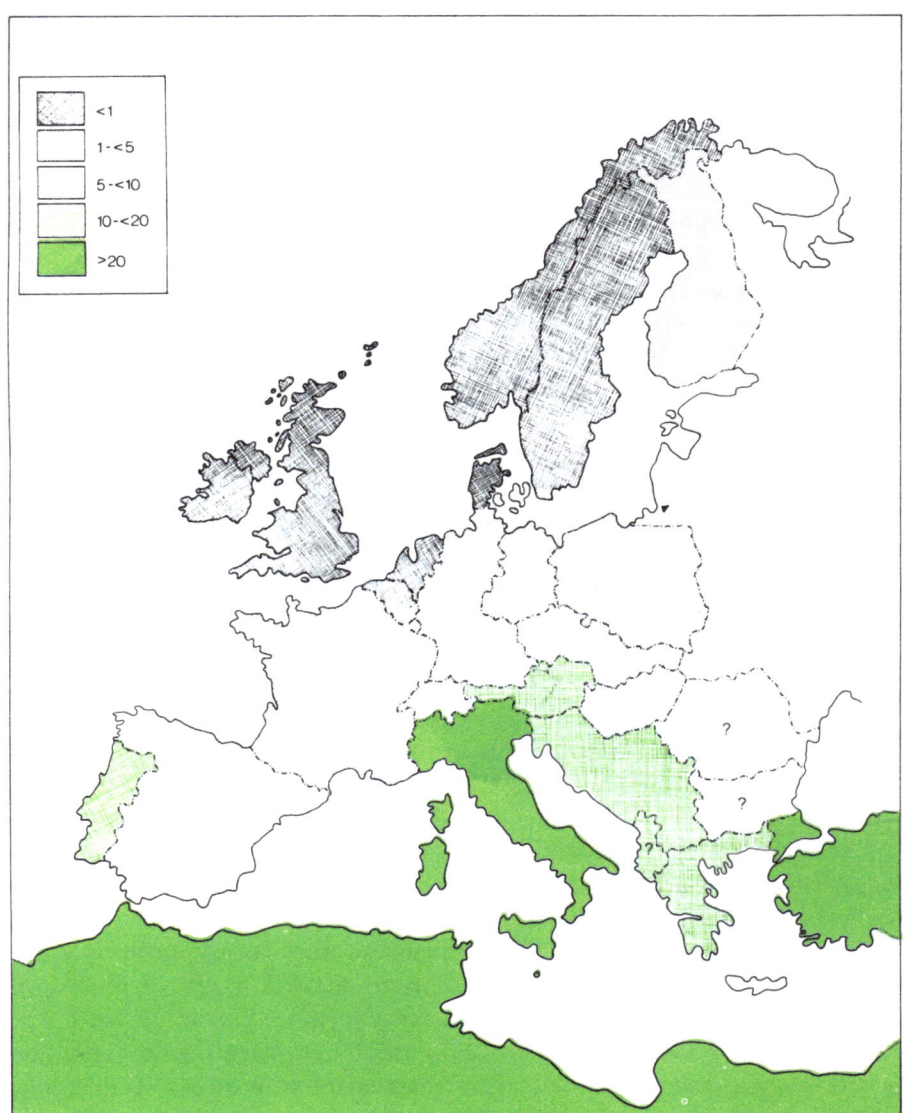

Figure 23. *Typhoid and paratyphoid fever reported during 1969 (*WHO*). Rates per 100,000 population.*

(1937), Zermatt (1963) and Aberdeen (1964). The incidence of typhoid in the UK is among the lowest in the world (Table 14), and the continuing source of sporadic cases of typhoid is mainly holidaymakers

Table 14. Cases of typhoid in the UK and the Republic of Ireland.

1973	104
1974	113
1975	165
1976	184
1977	206

and immigrants from endemic countries. Very occasionally sporadic infections may arise in individuals who have never been out of the country and the source of infection in such cases may be a chronic carrier in family or household contacts.

Prevention

The risk of acquiring typhoid abroad can be greatly reduced by the methods applicable to the prevention of cholera, i.e. avoiding uncooked vegetables and green salads, etc. and drinking bottled (preferably aerated) mineral water or water treated with sterilizing tablets.

Vaccine

Vaccine is the second line of defence. It is recommended (a) for travel to most areas outside Northern Europe, North America, Australia and New Zealand, (b) in the control of community or institutional outbreaks of typhoid fever, and (c) for family or other close contacts of a known typhoid carrier.

The type of vaccine used is similar to that used against cholera. Heat, alcohol or acetone are among the methods used to inactivate the bacteria.

There is no evidence of the efficacy of the paratyphoid A or B components of TAB vaccine, and a monovalent *S. typhi* vaccine or *S. typhi* combined with cholera and tetanus vaccine is recommended. The vaccine usually contains 1,000 million killed and preserved *S. typhi* and two doses are recommended at an interval of four to six weeks. The subcutaneous dose is usually 0.5 ml but reactions will be reduced if 0.1 ml is given intradermally.

A single dose will give some protection but it is unlikely that the vaccine will provide any protection until 10 to 20 days after immunisation. When it is not possible to give two doses separated by four weeks, three doses might be given at weekly intervals. Following a course of immunisation the vaccine should protect about 70 to 90 per cent of individuals against waterborne infections, but perhaps only about 40 per cent against food or drink which has been contaminated from infected water.

Reactions

Reactions after T or TAB vaccines are common and include swelling, redness and pain at the injection site. These usually occur within a few hours of injection and last for about two days. General reactions including fever, malaise, headache and nausea are often present for 24 to 48 hours. Other rare complications of the cardiovascular, renal and central nervous systems, etc. have been observed. TAB can cause endotoxic shock in antibody deficient patients. Reactions are reduced when the monovalent T vaccine is used, and further reduced when the intradermal route is employed.

Poliomyelitis

It is important to ensure that all travellers to countries outside Northern Europe, North America, Australia and New Zealand are immunised against poliomyelitis (see Chapter 7).

Virus Hepatitis

See Chapter 14.

Typhus Fever

Epidemic typhus is caused by *Rickettsia prowazekii*, which is transmitted from man to man by the body louse *Pediculus humanis corporis*. Man is the only reservoir of this rickettsia and he becomes infected by rubbing crushed infected lice or their faeces into wounds made by the bites of lice or into other abrasions. Infection may also occur by inhalation of dust contaminated by dried infected louse faeces.

Vaccine

The vaccine is prepared from formalin-inactivated *R. prowazekii* and is usually given as two primary subcutaneous injections four weeks apart followed by boosters at yearly intervals.

The vaccine is not recommended for travellers staying in urban accommodation in endemic countries. It could be of value to those who expect to be living in close personal contact with the indigenous population in places where the disease occurs, e.g. the mountainous areas of

Ethiopia, Rwanda, Burundi, Mexico, Ecuador, Bolivia, Peru and parts of Asia.

Plague

Plagus is a sylvatic enzootic infection of wild rodents in many parts of the world including the western USA and parts of Africa, Asia and South America. Plague may become epidemic if the domestic rat population becomes infected. The disease is caused by a bacterium *Yersinia pestis* which is usually transmitted by the flea *Xenopsylla cheopis* or by direct contact with infected rodents or humans.

Vaccine

The vaccine is prepared by inactivating *Y. pestis* with formalin. Plague vaccine is not generally recommended for travellers visiting endemic countries with the exception of Vietnam, Cambodia and Laos, unless their vocation or field work brings them into contact with wild rodents. The vaccine should be given intramuscularly in two or three spaced doses with boosters every six to twelve months while the individual remains in the endemic area.

13. Vaccines for Selective Use

Mumps

Mumps is spread by direct person-to-person contact by droplets from the upper respiratory passages, and man is the only known reservoir of the virus. Mumps is endemic in urban communities and is commoner in the winter months when upper respiratory tract infections are more frequent. The highest attack rate is in children between five and nine years of age. In the UK and North America about 30 to 40 per cent of adults who have not had mumps will have had a subclinical infection as evidenced by the presence of antibody. An attack of mumps results in life-long immunity.

Infection

As noted by Hippocrates about 2,000 years ago in Book I of the *Epidemics* the disease is more common in males than in females. In addition to infection of the salivary glands, other organs such as the CNS, testes, ovary, pancreas, etc. may be involved. These infections may occur without parotitis, at the same time as or before or after parotitis. With the exception of involvement of the CNS and testes, symptoms of infection of organs other than the salivary glands are rare.

Infection of the meninges may be fairly common but is usually symptomless. It may give rise to headache and bradycardia. Sometimes there may be signs and symptoms of aseptic meningitis (ASM) or meningoencephalitis, and mumps virus is one of the commonest viral causes of ASM. It may precede or accompany gland involvement. Complete recovery with no sequelae is usual but a number of patients may have a long convalescence with 'nervousness', occasional headache and muscle weakness. Nerve deafness is a rare complication.

Mumps virus may give rise to unilateral or bilateral orchitis, which is said to occur in about 20 per cent of postpubertal clinical infections. Even bilateral mumps orchitis very rarely leads to sterility.

Vaccine

In January 1968 a live attenuated mumps virus (the Jeryl Lynn strain, named after the child from whom it was isolated) was licensed in the United States. The 'wild' virus was attenuated by culture in embryonated hens' eggs and chick-embryo tissue culture. Vaccines prepared from that strain are said to be about 95 per cent effective. This is measured by the development of detectable antibody following the subcutaneous injection of approximately 5,000 $TCID_{50}$ in 0.5 ml. The levels of neutralizing antibody which develop are about one-fifth of the levels found after natural infection. Antibody persists for at least six years after vaccination and might be expected to be durable.

Who Should be Immunised?

Outside the USA there is little demand for routine vaccination against mumps and there seems no reason for its introduction for routine use. Mumps vaccine should certainly not be allowed to take priority over more essential community immunisation programmes. There may be a place for its selective use in children reaching puberty who have not had mumps. As already noted nearly half of such children may have had a subclinical infection, but it would be irrational to undertake serological studies to identify the susceptible individuals for immunisation and the mumps skin test is not a reliable indicator of immunity. There could be a place for its use in closed communities of children, basically to reduce the nuisance of an outbreak of mumps, and it might be introduced into such communities on the diagnosis of the first case.

Contraindications

Experience of the use of this vaccine is limited and the literature accompanying the vaccine should be consulted.

Rabies

Rabies is widely prevalent among various animal species throughout the world, except in the UK, Ireland, Scandinavia, Spain, Portugal, Cyprus, Australia, New Zealand, Hawaii and other Pacific Islands, and parts of the West Indies. The important animal reservoir in Europe includes foxes, badgers and wolves; in Africa it is the mongoose and jackal, and in the Americas the skunk, fox, racoon and fruit-eating bat. In Trinidad and South and Central America it is the vampire bat. (Other animal hosts are stoats, monkeys, deer and cattle which are essentially dead-end hosts.) In urban rabies dogs are the most important source of infection for man, and in many countries vaccination of dogs is compulsory. Rural rabies is a disease of wild biting animals, with sporadic disease among dogs and domestic animals. Man usually becomes infected by the bite of an infected animal for the virus is present in high titre in the saliva, but contact by licking may also transmit the disease. The incubation period depends on the site and severity of the bite for this determines the dose of virus introduced: it may be a few weeks after bites of the face and head, but may be up to six months after bites of the extremities.

In recent years wildlife rabies has been steadily increasing in the USA; in the UK, apart from two separate importations in monkeys in 1969 and 1970, there has been no rabies outside animal quarantine kennels, and the few fatal cases in man have all been infected abroad.

Control

This depends primarily on control of the animal hosts and vaccination of dogs in endemic countries.

Prevention in Man

Travellers in countries where rabies is present should avoid contact with wild animals and with domestic pets. This applies particularly to dogs and cats. Stray animals around camp sites (including puppies and kittens) should be avoided: docile and friendly animals may be suffering from 'dumb' rabies. If an individual is bitten the wound should be washed with soap and water. If the owner of the animal can be identified, information should be sought on the vaccination status of the animal because recently vaccinated animals rarely transmit rabies. In any event, immediate medical advice should be sought *locally* because the biting species may be known not to be infected, and the local doctor should be able to advise on immunisation.

Vaccine

Pasteur and rabies vaccine are practically synonymous. The most widely used modification of the Pasteur vaccine is inactivated rabbit-brain virus vaccine developed by Semple. Because of 'neuroparalytic accidents' following administration of this type of vaccine, efforts are now made to remove the encephalitogenic allergen by extracting the myelin with arcton.

Vaccines have also been developed by growing the virus in fertile duck eggs. This duck embryo vaccine (DEV) appears to produce fewer cases of allergic encephalitis but is less antigenic than the Semple vaccine. The factor producing allergic encephalitis appears to be absent from the brains of suckling mice less than 12 days old, and an inactive suckling mouse-brain-virus vaccine (SMBV) has been used extensively in South America and in the USSR. Vaccines made in diploid tissue culture have also been developed and look very hopeful but have not yet been tried on a sufficient scale for final evaluation.

Postexposure Immunisation

Postexposure immunisation is practical because of the long incubation period which usually follows infection, for the virus undergoes a period of local multiplication in muscle before spreading to the CNS by way of peripheral nerves. Such postexposure active immunisation may be accompanied by passive immunisation. The usual antiserum available is equine in origin and the dosage is 40 IU/kg bodyweight. This may give rise to allergic reactions and it is better to use specific rabies human immunoglobulin in a dose of 20 IU/kg which is free from reactions.

The treatment recommended by WHO for wounds involving possible exposure is shown in Tables 15 and 16.

Administration of the Vaccine

Because of reactions DEV is preferable, and 21 doses are given daily into the abdomen or lower back. When serum is given a delay of 24 hours is often recommended before starting the course of vaccine. Boosters are given 10, 20 and 40 days after completion of the course.

Where a reliable history is not available it is justifiable to modify the course and give a single dose of serum and three daily doses of vaccine. Provided the animal stays healthy for 10 days, no further vaccine should be required.

Evaluation of Vaccine

Each year about a million people throughout the world are given courses of rabies vaccines, but controlled studies of its effectiveness have never been made. One study in India indicated that 56 per cent of untreated exposed individuals developed rabies compared with seven per cent who had been vaccinated.

Pre-exposure Vaccination

Vaccination is recommended for those working in quarantine stations, veterinary surgeons, animal handlers, and travellers at high risk of contact with bats and wild animals. This does not mean that post-exposure immunisation can be omitted in the event of a known exposure of such immunised individuals.

DEV is given as two or three primary doses at monthly intervals, followed by a booster six months later. The immunity which develops should be confirmed by antibody studies and further doses of vaccine given if necessary. Satisfactory antibody levels may be achieved with the tissue culture vaccine in diploid cells; this is at present being studied.

Table 15. Local treatment of wounds involving possible exposure to rabies.

1. First-aid treatment
Since elimination of rabies virus at the site of infection by chemical or physical means is the most effective mechanism of protection, immediate washing and flushing with soap and water, detergent, or water alone is imperative (recommended procedure in all bite wounds including those unrelated to possible exposure to rabies). Then apply either 40–70 per cent alcohol, tincture or aqueous solutions of iodine, or 0.1 per cent quaternary ammonium compounds[1]

2. Treatment by or under direction of a physician
(a) Treat as above and then:
(b) Apply antirabies serum by careful instillation in the depth of the wound and by infiltration around the wound
(c) Postpone suturing of wound; if suturing is necessary use antiserum locally as stated above
(d) Where indicated, institute antitetanus procedures and administer antibiotics and drugs to control infections other than rabies

[1] Where soap has been used to clean wounds, all trace of it should be removed before the application of quaternary ammonium compounds because soap neutralizes the activity of such compounds.

Complications

Post-exposure immunisation with rabies vaccine may be followed by local reactions, constitutional symptoms and, as mentioned, allergic encephalitis. The exact rate of allergic encephalitis in such cases is difficult to estimate. In one study there were 50 neuroparalytic com-

Table 16. Specific systemic treatment.

Nature of exposure	Status of biting animal		Recommended treatment
	At time of exposure	During ten days[1]	
1. Contact, but no lesions indirect contact no contact	Rabid		None
2. Licks of the skin, scratches or abrasions, minor bites (covered areas of arms, trunk, and legs)	(a) Suspected as rabid[2]	Healthy	Start vaccine. Stop treatment if animal remains healthy for five days[1,3]
		Rabid	Start vaccine, administer serum upon positive diagnosis and complete the course of vaccine
	(b) Rabid, wild animal,[4] or animal unavailable for observation		Serum+vaccine
3. Licks of mucosa, major bites (multiple or on face, head, finger or neck)	Suspect[2] or rabid domestic or wild[4] animal, or animal unavailable for observation		Serum+vaccine. Stop treatment if animal remains healthy for five days[1,3]

[1] Observation period in this chart applies only to dogs and cats. Wild life should be killed and examined immediately because the incubation period in many wild animals may be very long.
[2] All unprovoked bites in endemic areas should be considered suspect unless proved negative by laboratory examination.
[3] Or if its brain is found negative by fluorescent antibody examination.
[4] In general, exposure to rodents and rabbits seldom, if ever, requires specific antirabies treatment.

plications following 100,218 courses of vaccine of Semple-type with a case fatality rate of 57 per cent. In a study of SMB vaccine the case fatality rate was 22 per cent and the number of neurological diseases in selected areas of South America was reduced from 51 in 1967 (an average of 30 per year from 1967 to 1971) to nine in 1972 when this vaccine was used. With DEV, the rate of neurological complications between 1958 and 1975 was about 4 per 100,000 vaccinated.

Anthrax

Anthrax is caused by a spore-bearing bacillus and is primarily a disease of herbivorous animals. Spores may remain alive for many years and have even been found in the so-called 'virgin' lands of Siberia. It is infrequent and sporadic in both the USA and UK. A human infection usually occurs as a cutaneous lesion—the so-called 'malignant pustule' which rarely contains pus. It has a haemorrhagic centre which becomes necrotic, giving rise to a black eschar.

The disease is essentially occupational and occurs in those exposed to infected hides and carcasses, and also to imported bonemeal, fishmeal and feedingstuffs.

Prevention depends on controlling anthrax in animals and by sterilizing imported hides, wool and hair. However, it is uneconomic to sterilize bonemeal and those handling it, e.g. warehousemen and gardeners, should be advised to wear gloves when doing so.

Vaccines

A vaccine is available for anyone subject to heavy exposure. It consists of an extract of *B. anthracis* and is given in a course of four intramuscular injections, each of 0.5 ml. The first three injections are given at three-weekly intervals and the fourth about six months later. Reinforcing doses should be given at about yearly intervals.

Typhus and Plague

In addition to their very occasional use for travellers (see Chapter 12), plague and typhus vaccines may be used for those at special risk. Typhus vaccine is recommended for medical personnel in areas where epidemic typhus occurs, laboratory personnel working with *Rickettsia prowazekii* and field workers in endemic countries. Plague vaccine is recommended for field workers and all laboratory personnel working with *Y. pestis* or with plague-infected rodents or fleas.

14. Passive Immunisation

It will be recalled that with passive immunisation immunity is achieved by injecting antibodies from another host. The onset of the protection is immediate and its duration depends on the titre of antibodies in the donor serum. Passive immunisation may be used therapeutically to provide protection until the host has developed antibodies naturally, or to prevent an infection for which active immunisation is neither indicated nor available.

Natural Passive Immunity

In the case of natural passive immunity, IgG is transferred across the placenta from the mother's plasma and the IgG is normally broken down with a half-life of about three to four weeks. For all practical purposes the duration of protection is about six to nine months in normal babies. In premature infants the transferred antibody may be below the level which will protect: it may be augmented artificially by the injection of immunoglobulins.

Artificial Passive Immunity

In artificial passive immunity the injection of immunoglobulins produces immediate protection and there is obviously no lag phase nor any secondary response if further injections of the immunoglobulins are made. In fact, when immunoglobulins from a foreign host are injected they are catabolized like any other protein, or used in reactions with the antigens of the invading organism. Normally antibodies to foreign immunoglobulins will develop about 10 to 14 days after injection but if the host has had previous experience with the foreign immunoglobulin the antibodies to it will develop more quickly and the 'serum' will be rapidly eliminated. This presented a problem when horse antitetanus serum (ATS) was used in the prophylaxis of tetanus, for any repeated injection of horse serum often caused such rapid production of antibody against it, that the ATS antitoxin was removed from the circulation and rendered ineffective long before it had had any chance to protect the patient. The combination of horse serum with precipitating antibody in the tissues may lead to serum sickness (hypersensitivity type 3), or to anaphylactic shock (hypersensitivity type 1) and death. These properties of horse and other animal sera have led to its virtual abandonment for use in passive immunisation and human immunoglobulin has taken its place. Theoretically different classes of human immunoglobulins could elicit antigen–antibody reactions, but because they are homologous they do not excite the type of antibody response elicited by foreign animal proteins. If human immunoglobulins are inoculated intravenously, they may produce severe reactions because of aggregations of antibody molecules which react with complement.

Normal Immunoglobulin

The immunoglobulins in common use are prepared from pools of human plasma or placental blood. The immunoglobulin prepared from normal sources was called *gammaglobulin*, but it is now referred to as *human normal immunoglobulin* in Britain and *immune serum globulin* (*human*) in the USA. In the preparation of human normal immunoglobulin, the plasma from at least 1,000 donors is used for each batch, thus all batches will have comparable levels of the antibodies prevalent in the donor community. Protective antibodies to all infectious diseases will not be represented in preparations of immunoglobulin for normal immunoglobulin contains mainly IgG which is not generally effective against, for example, invasive bacteria. Immunoglobulins are in general of value only in those bacterial diseases which stimulate antitoxins and in virus infections, particularly those which produce a viraemia and to which immunity is largely mediated by circulating antibody.

In the UK normal immunoglobulin is prepared as a 15 g per cent solution in two sizes of vial: 250 mg in 1.7 ml solution, and 750 mg in 5.1 ml solution. Doses are usually prescribed by weight of immunoglobulin. In the USA immune serum globulin contains 165 mg of gammaglobulin per ml, and consists of most of the antibodies in plasma concentrated about 25 times. Doses are given in ml/kg of body weight.

127

Specific Immunoglobulin

The second type of human immunoglobulin available was in the past referred to as *hyperimmune gammaglobulin* or convalescent gammaglobulin. This contains increased amounts of antibody to specific diseases (e.g. smallpox and tetanus) and is now called *human specific immunoglobulin* in Britain and *special immune serum globulin* in the USA. The specific names of these preparations are human antivaccine or human antitetanus immunoglobulin in the UK and vaccinia or tetanus immune globulin (human) in the USA. Specific immunoglobulins are prepared by pooling the blood of convalescent patients or by bleeding immunised donors whose antibody has recently been boosted by immunisation.

In the UK specific immunoglobulins are prepared as solutions with a protein content of not less than 10 g or more than 15 g per cent. The immunoglobulins are suspended in saline and give a clear yellowish or slightly brown fluid which should be stored at +4° C. (They may develop a slight turbidity on storage.)

In the UK human immunoglobulins are prepared at the Blood Products Laboratory, Lister Institute of Preventive Medicine (Elstree) and at the Plasma Fraction Centre, Edinburgh. In England and Wales they are available through the Public Health Laboratory Service Laboratories with exception of human antitetanus immunoglobulin, which is kept at a number of designated centres and is also obtainable commercially (Imutet BW). In Scotland normal and specific immunoglobulins are available at regional transfusion centres. Two vial sizes are available: 250 mg and 500 mg. In Britain the supply of specific immunoglobulin depends on the co-operation of general practitioners, and there is need for antivaricella/zoster, antitetanus and to a lesser extent antimumps, antiherpes simplex and antirubella specific immunoglobulins. Patients who have suffered an attack of one of these diseases (except tetanus) in the previous three months should be asked to donate some blood, as should any adult who has recently been reimmunised against tetanus or smallpox. The names and addresses of anyone volunteering to do so should be sent to the director of the local blood transfusion centre. Supplies of these specific immunoglobulins can only be prepared if such donations of blood are forthcoming.

In the USA the specific immunoglobulins contain about 10 to 20 times the levels of antibody in pools of 'normal' donor sera. As with immune serum globulin, doses in the USA are given in ml per kg body weight. Vaccinia immune globulin (VIG) may be obtained within a few hours in the USA by contacting one of the designated consultants listed by the Regional Blood Centers of the American Red Cross; otherwise these special immunoglobulins are obtainable commercially.

When immunoglobulins are injected, the initial concentration of antibody in the preparation becomes diluted by the recipient's body fluids to a dilution of plasma equal to about eight per cent of the recipient's bodyweight. Antibodies which are present in the immunoglobulins in low titre (e.g. rubella) could thus be diluted below a level which on theoretical grounds would be expected to be effective. Because of this dilution factor it is obvious that the weight: dose ratio in the use of immunoglobulins is important.

Immunoglobulins should always be injected intramuscularly. Reaction is rare although sometimes there is slight pain at the site of injection.

They must *never* be injected intravenously, because this may produce serious reactions such as tachycardia, pallor and a sense of pressure in the chest and pain in the flank.

Diphtheria

Diphtheria is one of the very few diseases for which antitoxin prepared in animals is still used. The efficacy of this antitoxin and the disappearance of the disease following immunisation with toxoid make the study of the use of human antidiphtheria immunoglobulin virtually irrelevant.

Antitoxin prepared in horses (which, early on, became the animals of choice) was introduced by Roux at the Pasteur Institute at the end of the last century after the discovery of passive immunity by Behring and his colleagues in Berlin. Its use probably reduced the case fatality rate of diphtheria from about 40 per cent to less than 10 per cent. It soon became obvious that some measurement of the amount of antibody in the immunoglobulin was required. This led to the whole concept of standardization not only of sera but of other biological fluids and to the subsequent establishment of many international standards.

For therapy antidiphtheria serum has to be given immediately the clinical diagnosis is made and is said to be 100 per cent effective if given within 24 hours of the onset. As a prophylactic in the control of outbreaks in the UK, ADS is now confined to closed institutions such as homes for the mentally subnormal where outbreaks should normally be prevented by active immunisation and boosting. After a case has been diagnosed in an institute all contacts and any home contacts should be swabbed (nose and throat). The immunisation status of these contacts should be investigated by the Schick test. The amount of toxin in the test dose is adequate to boost the immunity of Schick-negative individuals. All Schick-positive individuals should be given an injection of toxoid in a form such as PTAP (purified toxin absorbed on aluminium phosphate) and at the same time 500 units of antitoxin. This antitoxin may give rise to general reactions in about five to eight per cent of individuals. However, when diphtheria was prevalent it was believed that the risk of diphtheria in the non-immunised was greater than the risk of sensitization to horse serum. All contacts should be kept under close surveillance for three to four days until the laboratory results on isolations become available. All individuals who are non-immune should be given a second dose of PTAP four to six weeks later. There is no experience of how the availability of penicillin and erythromycin might modify this regime today.

Reactions

If horse serum or other animal sera are injected, it must be understood that there are no entirely satisfactory tests for hypersensitivity to animal sera. The greatest reliance on the likelihood of a hypersensitivity reaction should be placed on whether or not the individual has ever been given an injection of animal serum, and whether or not there is any family history of allergic conditions. If there is no experience or history of hypersensitivity, an intramuscular injection of the serum may be given and the patient kept under observation for at least 30 minutes (although serum sickness may develop seven to 10 days later). If the patient has been given animal serum, he should be given a trial dose of 0.2 ml of serum and observed for 30 minutes. If there is no reaction the rest of the dose of serum may be given intramuscularly. If there *is* a reaction the serum should be given in 0.2 ml vol. by the subcutaneous route at intervals of 30 minutes until the total dose has been injected.

Patients with an allergic history appear to be at greatest risk of developing severe reactions to foreign sera. In their case 0.2 ml of the serum should be diluted 1:10 in distilled water and given subcutaneously, and the patient should be kept under observation for 30 minutes. If there is no reaction 0.2 ml of the undiluted serum may be given subcutaneously, and if there is no subsequent reaction the remainder of the total dose may be given by the intramuscular route. If there is a reaction the remainder of the serum should be given in 0.2 ml volumes half-hourly preceded by a dose of a quick-acting antihistamine before the injections are started.

At all times adrenaline (1:1,000) and hydrocortisone hemisuccinate should be available for immediate use in case a reaction occurs.

The intravenous injection of serum should not be used except by those experienced with its dangers, and its use should be limited to hospital practice.

Tetanus

As already mentioned (Chapter 4) the prevention of tetanus depends on active immunisation of all children with tetanus toxoid, with boosters at school entry and at school leaving and further boosters to adults at high risk. The prophylaxis of tetanus in immunised individuals who suffer wounds or burns has also been discussed and briefly their basic immunity may be boosted with tetanus toxoid.

Since reactions occur after the use of animal sera the use of horse serum for the prophylaxis of tetanus was virtually abandoned by many practitioners even before human antitetanus immunoglobulin became available.

The use of ATS is now essentially of historical interest in developed countries for the management of wounds or burns in persons who have not been actively immunised. ATS has been replaced by human antitetanus immunoglobulin. This is prepared from the plasma of selected donors whose plasma level of tetanus antitoxin has been boosted by a recent dose of toxoid. Human antitetanus immunoglobulin may be in relatively short supply from government sources, but it is also available commercially. In the treatment of clean wounds (with minimal tissue damage sustained in circumstances unlikely to involve contamination with tetanus spores, such as a cut with a razor or by glass), provided that the patient receives medical attention within six hours of the trauma, cleansing and suture and an injection of 0.5 ml adsorbed tetanus toxoid should be recommended, with completion of the course of toxoid as required. With other wounds or burns (with the exception of those listed below) it is usually recommended that in addition to tetanus toxoid and adequate cleansing of the wound, penicillin by injection preferably as a mixture of benzathine, procaine and benzyl-penicillin in the proportions of 2:1:1, to cover for at least four days should be given and 0.5 ml adsorbed toxoid. Subsequently the course of tetanus toxoid should be completed. For patients sensitive to penicillin, tetracycline in doses of 250 mg six-hourly for four days may be used.

The experts recommend that human antitetanus immunoglobulin

should be used selectively in addition to wound toilet, penicillin, etc. and toxoid, for non-immunised persons who have:

1. Sustained a wound or burn more than six hours before attending for treatment.

2. Wounds which are likely to be infected with tetanus organisms because of contamination with soil, manure, etc.

3. Wounds which are septic or contain devitalized tissues.

4. Puncture wounds.

The dose is 250 IU given intramuscularly. The preparations usually available contain not less than 50 IU/ml.

In 1965, the Department of Health and Social Security in England and Wales agreed (for medicolegal reasons) that ATS could be used at the discretion of the doctor concerned, and presumably a similar proviso will cover the use of human antitetanus immunoglobulin.

The importance of completing a course of tetanus toxoid after receiving wounds cannot be stressed too emphatically.

Other Animal Sera

Although potent antisera can be prepared in horses against the organisms of gas gangrene (*Clostridium welchii*, *Cl. oedematiens* and *Cl. septicum*), they are rarely used in prophylaxis. Similarly, passive immunisation with immunoglobulins against the toxins of *Cl. botulinum* seems to have limited value.

Virus Diseases
Normal Immunoglobulin

In addition to containing antibodies to those 'wild' viruses which are circulating in the community, human normal immunoglobulin will presumably also contain antibodies to viral antigens contained in commonly used vaccines (assuming that the viral antigens stimulate reasonable levels of durable circulating antibody).

Human normal immunoglobulin has been shown to be effective for the prevention of measles, infective hepatitis (hepatitis A) and in certain cases of chickenpox. It is of less use in rubella and poliomyelitis.

Measles

Normal immunoglobulin should contain not less than 50 IU measles antibody per ml. Since the 1940s it has been known to modify or prevent measles and was used widely for this purpose before the introduction of measles vaccine.

The problem of attenuating measles should not arise in babies under six months of age, unless they are premature since, at present, nearly all normal babies have maternally transmitted measles antibodies which are usually effective for at least the first six months of life. The dosage recommended in such cases when given not more than one week after exposure is 250 mg (0.05 ml/kg body-weight in the USA). For prevention, the use of immunoglobulin is essentially limited to the few babies in whom an attack of measles must be avoided, e.g. the small chronically ill baby with respiratory or cardiac disease who, if exposed to measles infection, could be tided over the infection and actively immunised at a convenient time. In such cases immunisation should be attempted as soon as possible after exposure. The recommended dose in the UK for infants is 250 mg and for children one to two years and three years and over, 500 and 750 mg respectively. The dose in the USA is 0.25 ml/kg of body weight. This method of prevention decreases in effectiveness the longer the delay after exposure and after four days it is likely that only attenuation of the infection will be achieved.

Human normal immunoglobulin has also been used to modify the reactions of measles vaccine, e.g. in children suffering from chronic diseases of the heart or lungs. In the UK supplies for this purpose are held by local authorities. Each vial contains four to eight IU measles antibody in 15 mg immunoglobulin (in the form of 0.5 ml 3 g per cent solution). The optimum dose for modification of reactions is about 0.6 mg per lb body weight. It is important not to exceed this dose because excess immunoglobulin may inhibit the multiplication of measles vaccine virus. A vial thus contains sufficient immunoglobulin for a child in the second year of life. The dose of immunoglobulin is given at the same time as the measles vaccine in the opposite limb.

Infective Hepatitis (Hepatitis A)

Many studies have shown the value of normal immunoglobulin in the prevention and control of clinical manifestations of infective hepatitis. It is of particular value in controlling infection in contacts in mental and other closed institutions, such as children's homes, where the risk of spread of the disease is great. It has also been recommended under certain conditions in ordinary schools and in the protection of home contacts, particularly pregnant women.

It should be given as early as possible after exposure but it still appears to prevent the clinical illness if given as late as 14 days after exposure. Individuals who have been passively immunised may develop jaundice within the first two weeks after injection of immunoglobulin, presumably because it has been given too late in the incubation period of the infection. It is effective in preventing clinical disease in about 85 per cent of contacts. In the UK the recommended dose is 250 mg for children under 10 years of age and 500 mg for those of 10 years or more. In the USA 0.02 ml per kg of body weight is recommended. It is obvious that the use of gammaglobulin in the control of infection among contacts varies greatly from one situation to another and depends on the degree and nature of the contact.

Normal immunoglobulin is also recommended for travellers visiting countries where the risk of infection is great, i.e. where hygiene is poor and where there are considerable opportunities for faecal–oral contamination. Such countries are obviously included in the continents of Africa, Asia and South America. The recommendation in the UK is to give a dose of 750 mg immunoglobulin which usually confers protection for is at least six months and many individuals may get a subclinical infection under cover of the immunoglobulin which should provide a durable immunity. A traveller who has never had infective hepatitis should be given a second injection of immunoglobulin after six months if he remains in the country where the chance of infection is great.

In the USA, immunoglobulin is not recommended for travellers on ordinary tourist routes for less than three months; for longer journeys 0.02 ml/kg of body weight is recommended and 0.05 ml/ body weight for travellers planning to stay three months or more in tropical areas or in developing countries where hepatitis A is common and hygiene poor.

Chickenpox

Chickenpox can be a severe disease with a 20 per cent mortality in the neonatal period for infants with no maternal antibody. Normal immunoglobulin may be of some value in modifying such infections in newborn babies known not to have maternal antibody, and in premature and other abnormal babies under six months of age if it is given within three days of exposure.

It would also seem reasonable to give immunoglobulin to a neonate whose mother had developed chickenpox in the last two weeks of pregnancy.

Normal immunoglobulin may also be given for the attenuation of chickenpox in eczematous and other ill children, in pregnant women and in patients on steroids or immunosuppressive drugs. It will not prevent chickenpox (see specific antivaricella immunoglobulin).

Poliomyelitis

Although human normal immunoglobulin contains antibodies in adequate titre to prevent poliomyelitis, its use is rarely indicated in the control of poliomyelitis in view of the effectiveness of vaccination. In any event the uncertainty of the time of exposure to infection presents a practical difficulty in its effective use.

Rubella

Normal immunoglobulin should confer protection against rubella if given before exposure. However, in practice normal immunoglobulin cannot regularly be considered to be of practical value in the prevention of congenital defects in women who have been exposed to rubella during pregnancy. There are two reasons for this. First, patients with rubella may be infectious for about a week before the rash appears, and thus susceptible contacts may be infected and already have a viraemia before it is appreciated that infection has occurred. It is then too late to expect normal immunoglobulin to have any effect. Second, it seems that the quantity of antibody to rubella even in a large dose of normal immunoglobulin is insufficient to neutralize the virus consistently. At the same time there is a suggestion from many studies that normal immunoglobulin might fractionally reduce the incidence of congenital defects in pregnant women exposed to rubella. It is worth remembering that a high proportion of mothers (as high as 90 per cent in some areas) have natural circulating rubella antibody and obviously it would be unnecessary even to consider giving such mothers immunoglobulin.

There might be a case for giving immunoglobulin to a known susceptible pregnant woman who is a contact of a contact, and whose pregnancy cannot be terminated following an infection. Thus if a mother heard that her child had been a contact of a patient with rubella, an immediate dose of immunoglobulin might protect her from infection when her own child became infectious.

If, after an injection of normal immunoglobulin, the signs and symptoms of rubella do not occur in an exposed susceptible woman, this cannot give complete assurance that infection and viraemia had been prevented and that fetal damage had not occurred.

Human Specific Immunoglobulins

Rubella

High-titre immunoglobulin given in high doses within 24 hours of viral exposure has been shown to be effective in preventing viraemia in rubella infections, and there may be some cases where specific anti-rubella immunoglobulin is indicated. As indicated the efficacy of immunoglobulin in rubella depends on the dose and titre of the IgG, the time of administration in relation to the time of exposure and the immune status of the woman.

Although the logistics are great and there are difficulties of preparing high titre specific immunoglobulin, further studies are clearly indicated in the use of specific antirubella immunoglobulin for the prevention of rubella in selected susceptible pregnant women where termination of pregnancy cannot be carried out if infection occurs. It might be worth testing its value in the pregnant contact of the contact referred to above.

Vaccinia

Human antivaccinia immunoglobulin is prepared from blood collected three to four weeks after revaccination. It is therefore important that the need for such blood should be explained to individuals undergoing vaccinations and that they should be encouraged to volunteer as donors. Antivaccinia immunoglobulin should contain not less than 500 IU antibody per ml.

It is used for the prevention and treatment of the complications of smallpox vaccination and for the prevention of smallpox in contacts. Thus when vaccination is necessary in the presence of contraindications, e.g. in persons with eczema or on steroid therapy, a dose of antivaccinia immunoglobulin should be given in the opposite arm at the same time as vaccination. (The vaccination site should be examined in about a week to ensure that the vaccination has 'taken'.) Again, if vaccination is essential for a pregnant woman antivaccinia immunoglobulin may be given at the same time as vaccination. Antivaccinia immunoglobulin is also of value for any individual who has been accidentally vaccinated. In the case of an eye infection a one per cent solution of immunoglobulin may be instilled into the conjunctival sac.

In all familial or other unvaccinated close contacts exposed to smallpox, antivaccinia immunoglobulin is indicated in addition to vaccination. It is of particular importance in contacts who have not been vaccinated within 24 or 48 hours of exposure. The dose recommended in the USA is 0.3 ml/kg of body weight (see p. 50); those proposed in the UK are given in Table 17.

It might rationally be assumed that antivariola immunoglobulin would be more effective and this could be prepared from donors who had recovered from smallpox in countries where the disease has been endemic. The almost total global eradication of smallpox makes this hardly worth further consideration, but the existence of a reserve of antivaccinia immunoglobulin is important.

Hepatitis Type B (Serum Hepatitis)

Plasma of individuals possessing antibody to the Australia (hepatitis B surface) antigen (HBsA) is used to prepare specific anti-HBsA immunoglobulin. The value of this specific immunoglobulin for preventing hepatitis B is at present being investigated. It would appear that this immunoglobulin can confer considerable protection after accidental contamination and also if given before exposure. Its large-scale use for high-risk groups such as the staff of haemodialysis units is less certain.

Chickenpox and Zoster

Antivaricella/zoster (v-z) immunoglobulin prepared from individuals convalescent from chickenpox or herpes zoster might be expected to confer passive immunity more effectively than normal immunoglobulin. In appropriate doses it will usually prevent varicella if given within three days of exposure. Its main value, however, is in individuals with immunological abnormalities, e.g. those being treated with steroids or immunosuppressive drugs, or those who have leukaemia or other neoplastic diseases in whom an infection with v-z virus might otherwise be a progressive and fatal disease. Specific immunoglobulin could also be of value to prevent cross-infection with chickenpox in children's wards, and to control and prevent death from neonatal infections with varicella in babies with blood dyscrasias and chronic illnesses.

It will always be relatively scarce because it can be prepared only from the plasma of adults convalescent from chickenpox or herpes zoster. Such people are urgently required as donors. So far supplies have been insufficient to assess its value. The recommended doses of antizoster immunoglobulin are given in Table 17.

Herpes Simplex

The value of specific antiherpes simplex immunoglobulin has not yet been adequately studied because of the shortage of supply. It might

Table 17. Recommended doses of antivaccinia immunoglobulin for smallpox and of antizoster immunoglobulin for chickenpox and herpes zoster.

Age in years	Dose (mg)
Under 1	500
1–6	1,000
7–14	1,500
15 and over	2,000

be of value for treating some cases of disseminated herpes simplex infections.

Rabies

Human antirabies immunoglobulin can be prepared only from the blood of those who have been actively immunised against rabies, otherwise animal immune sera are used (see Chapter 13).

Other Conditions

In addition to the possible use of immunoglobulin for premature babies and in antibody deficient syndromes its use can always be considered for any conditions where antibody production is suppressed or reduced.

Conclusion

Before passive immunisation can be fully exploited those preparing the human immunoglobulins must have the fullest co-operation of physicians to encourage those who have recovered from certain virus diseases or have been recently immunised to donate blood.

15. Immunisation in Tropical Environments

Vaccines are no substitute for general improvements in socioeconomic conditions for the control of infectious diseases. Even with the most advanced medical technology, immunisation by itself is unlikely to compensate for adverse effects of environmental and behavioural factors. It will produce poor and disappointing results unless it is accompanied by control of the source of infection, breaking the chain of transmission and increasing the resistance of the host. It should be developed as part of a programme for improving health care and health education and not in isolation.

Socioeconomic Factors

In many developing countries the urban immunisation programme will have similar schedules to those in developed countries. The main problem, however, is the administration of vaccination programmes and the delivery of vaccine in rural communities. First of all an order of priority of diseases to be prevented has to be decided. Data on the importance of a disease come from two sources: from what governments consider their main health problems (which are often based on general impressions) and from the principal causes of death. In developing countries this type of information does not very often include the specific fevers of childhood for which vaccines are available.

Notifications

At present the notification of infectious diseases is inevitably less accurate in the tropical environment than in developed countries. When it is recalled how unreliable was the reporting of smallpox at the beginning of the global eradication programme one must not expect the notifications of a disease like poliomyelitis to be very informative when there is no interest or advantage in reporting the disease.

Good notifications are essential for the planning of any immunisation programme and its surveillance. In many developing countries notifications can be improved by progressively increasing the completeness and regularity of weekly reports from all fixed medical units throughout the country including the sending of nil returns.

Improved Socioeconomic Conditions

In Chapter 5 it was mentioned that over the years the decline in notifications and mortality from measles and from whooping cough in England and Wales was perhaps more dependent on improved socioeconomic conditions and family size than on immunisation. A similar story exists for tuberculosis. The great reduction of tuberculosis in some developed countries has been largely dependent on better social conditions rather than on vaccine. The decline in mortality from that disease in the middle of the 19th century in the UK probably owed less to specific measures of preventing the disease in the individual than to the general improvement in the standard of living (such as better nutrition and better hygiene). The importance of improved environmental conditions, family planning and health education may have to have precedence when it comes to considering extensive immunisation programmes.

Vaccines

Consideration must be given to the overall cost benefit of vaccines compared with general measures in the control of infectious disease. In May 1974 the 27th WHO World Assembly promulgated a resolution committing WHO to an Expanded Programme of Immunisation. In the light of the immense influence of uncontrolled population growth on health, it is questionable whether any wide-scale immunisation programmes in the developing countries—apart from that involved in the global control of smallpox—are justified. However, the majority opinion favours them and considers that the available vaccines must be used hand in hand with other public health measures. It has been suggested that if deaths in children are prevented by immunisation there will be more reason for adopting family planning proposals than waiting for an infectious disease such as measles to act as a postnatal birth control weapon.

Most countries in the Third World have some kind of immunisation programme and many of those in North America have had organized programmes for many years. However, at present 90 per cent or more of the susceptible children in the developing world are not being immunised.

While decisions on any immunisation programme must be based on national resources, consideration must be given to the needs of the community. In part this must be based on their beliefs and culture which may not necessarily be reflected by the prevalence of the disease in urban hospitals for the needs of a rural community cannot be extrapolated from urban data.

The vaccines generally recommended for use in tropical countries are smallpox, BCG, dip/tet/pert (sometimes combined with typhoid), measles, poliomyelitis, and yellow fever for those at high risk to that disease (Figure 22).

Smallpox

Smallpox has had pride of place because it threatened the developed countries and because it was possible to eradicate it. (The global eradication of that disease is discussed in Chapter 6.)

Tuberculosis

Tuberculosis is probably the most pressing problem in the developing countries. The efficacy of BCG in these countries was greatly influenced by the introduction of freeze-dried vaccine and the multiple puncture technique. The potential of jet injectors does not seem to have been realized, for they have given irregular performances (probably because of lack of effective maintenance). The development of simple techniques for administering BCG, e.g. with the bifurcated needle, has so far been disappointing but should be pursued.

The cost of BCG is small—about two cents (USA) per dose—when purchased in bulk. About 14 cents per dose must be added to the cost of the vaccine for delivery and other indirect costs (as estimated from the West and Central African smallpox eradication programmes). It has been estimated that the cost of treating a tuberculous child in hospital in Uganda could provide BCG for 7,000 individuals and give them 80 per cent protection for presumably at least 10 years and possibly some protection against leprosy.

In those countries which have an existing BCG immunisation programme it would seem sensible to try to graft other routine immunisations on to it and expand it step by step throughout the country.

Diphtheria/Tetanus/Pertussis/Typhoid

The prevalence of diphtheria, tetanus or pertussis in developing countries is not well known nor is the extent of the demand or need for triple vaccine (DPT). In those countries with a high incidence of tetanus neonatorum, all girls should certainly be given a course of immunisation with tetanus toxoid at some time.

In countries with a high incidence of enteric fever, typhoid vaccine may be combined with the triple vaccine, but the use of typhoid vaccine although sometimes less costly is secondary to health education and efforts to improve water supplies. The cost of DPT with or without typhoid vaccine is about 15 cents (USA) for three doses. About one-third of the dose given by the intradermal route will produce the same antigenic response as a full dose given subcutaneously. This not only reduces reactions and cost but also provides a useful marker at the site of injection for some time.

Poliomyelitis

Many administrators do not consider that poliomyelitis is a priority disease in the tropical environment. It would seem that this depends on what is being measured, for a hopeless cripple is surely more uneconomic than a dead child. In any event the survival of a severely handicapped child in underdeveloped countries must be very limited.

The cost of oral poliovirus vaccine (OPV) is about 15 cents (USA) per dose of trivalent vaccine. OPV is often said to be less effective (as measured by circulating antibodies) in tropical and subtropical countries than in temperate ones, either because of interference by other enteroviruses in the gut or from inhibitory properties of breast milk. There is no good evidence to show that interference is of special importance in tropical climates nor that breast milk influences vaccine 'takes'. The suggestion that breast feeding should be withheld six hours prior to and following a dose of OPV because of the supposed inhibitory effect of milk on the viruses is not supported by present laboratory studies.

In an attempt to explain the lower rate of antibody conversion following immunisation with OPV in some tropical countries it has been suggested that babies in these countries do not always develop detectable circulating antibody after infection with polioviruses because of their nutritional state. Poliomyelitis may have a high attack rate in small babies in developing countries because in general antibody which has developed in girls following infection in childhood may never reach a very high level. When such girls have babies the maternal antibody which they transmit may be of such low titre that it rapidly falls below an effective protective level. The baby is then susceptible to poliomyelitis in the first few months of life as compared with children in other parts of the world who may have protection from maternal antibody for a considerable time during the first year.

As with all vaccines there must be continuous surveillance of OPV and it *must* be ensured that all vaccines made available for immunisation programmes in developing countries comply in all details with the WHO requirements or their equivalent.

It would seem more sensible to base studies on the efficacy of poliovirus vaccines on paralytic attack rates than on antibody surveys.

Measles

In some developing countries measles is the commonest infectious disease of childhood and its severity is related to the state of nutrition of the child. It is not the virus which may make the mortality in a malnourished child 400 times greater than in a well-nourished child, but the culture and the diet of the community. In some places the mortality from measles closely parallels that of kwashiorkor and measles is probably the commonest precipitating factor of protein malnutrition in developing countries. Reduction of malnutrition could have a very great effect on measles mortality and reduction of measles would reduce the effects of malnutrition.

More mistakes are being made in measles vaccination programmes than have been seen with any other vaccine. No programme should be initiated without consideration of the long-range implications. There is no place for the 'big bang' campaign and immunisation against measles should be integrated with other immunisations, health education, maternal and child welfare and family planning programmes. Because of the younger age of infection with measles and the high birth rate in developing countries, vaccination against measles, if undertaken, should as far as possible be carried out at about nine months of age.

Not only is measles vaccine expensive to buy (30 US cents per dose) but like poliovirus vaccine it is expensive to store and to deliver because of the 'cold chain' which is required from the deep freeze in the medical

143

store to the rural dispensary or mobile immunisation team. An example of this problem was highlighted in data from an analysis of a measles immunisation campaign in the Cameroons. This showed that 83 per cent of the vaccine was wasted. Thus 44 per cent of the children were immune to measles and 1.4 per cent were too young or too old at the time of the campaign; 25 per cent of the vaccine administered was impotent because of loss of titre, etc. due to tropical conditions and 12.6 per cent of the vaccine was thrown away. Because of these problems an effective inactivated vaccine could be a great advantage, and perhaps in the future a polyvalent inactivated virus mixture might, in a single shot, immunise against the majority of common childhood diseases (see p. 65).

Schedules of Immunisation

In 1976 in the developing world 60 million children reached one year of age but very little work seems to be in progress to establish the optimum schedules and age for their immunisation.

In establishing any schedule it is desirable to immunise just before the age of highest morbidity. This can be more readily and accurately ascertained by information on age-specific attack rates than by serological tests. In general, since most infectious diseases occur at an earlier age in developing countries than in industrialized ones, the age for commencing immunisation should be younger in the former.

The schedules which have often been recommended for developing countries in past years have usually followed those introduced into Europe and North America, with little rationale except that they were effective. Schedules at static health centres have often followed some scheme such as that outlined in Table 18, but experience in many countries has shown that such schedules result in very low proportions of completed immunisations. A much simpler schedule is shown in Table 19, which although it probably does not ensure such a high probability of individual protection as the schedule in Table 17, might achieve a greater community effect by obtaining greater acceptance if the schedule is completed.

Experience in many tropical countries has shown that vaccination coverage declines sharply in persons living no more than two or three miles from health centres. However, it is possible to vaccinate 80 to 90 per cent of the population in such areas by using mobile teams based on health centres.

It seems likely that for effective immunisation of rural populations

Table 18. Typical schedule of immunisation.

1–3 months	4–8 months	9–12 months	5–6 years
Dip/tet/pert typhoid BCG (or at birth)	Dip/tet/pert typhoid	Measles	Dip/tet/pert typhoid
Polio	Polio	Polio Yellow fever	

multiple antigen immunisation campaigns carried out annually by mobile teams will for many years be the method of choice. A simple schedule for such a team has been suggested, in which the mean height of children of 24 months of age in the area is used as the criterion for entry into the vaccination line (Figure 24). Children who passed the height test would be given DPT and OPV, those who could not walk would not be vaccinated, those who could, would be given their once only BCG, measles and in some places, smallpox vaccine. On the next and on all future visits they would be checked for BCG (or smallpox) scars. Those with a scar would receive only DPT and those with no scar BCG, measles and smallpox. Simple counts of those with scars from marker vaccines could indicate the success of the immunisation programme in any district.

The eventual success of any programme should not be measured by the number of doses of vaccine bought or delivered but by the effect of the programme on the incidence of the disease and achievement of community requirements.

Surveillance

Surveillance is all important. It has been stressed that data collected

Table 19. A simplified schedule of immunisation suggested for use in developing countries.

1–3 months	Under 6 months	Over 12 months
Dip/tet/pert Polio BCG (as marker)	Dip/tet/pert Polio Measles Smallpox (as marker)	Dip/tet/pert Polio

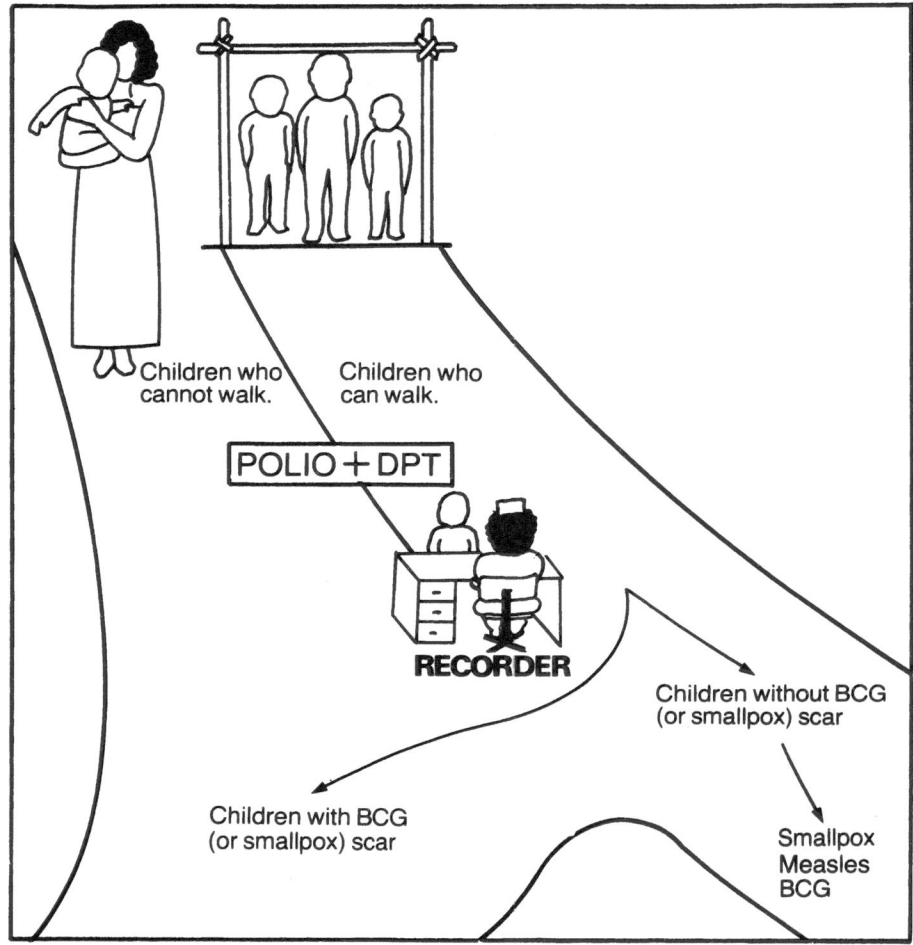

Figure 24. *Simple schedule for routine immunisation in rural areas.*

for surveillance should be used to modify or expand programmes. If surveillance of a disease is to be successful it must lead to action. From experience with smallpox surveillance it has been suggested that notifications might profitably be restricted to those diseases for which intervention would be implemented if the incidence reached some defined level or in which some form of continuing programme of immunisation is in progress.

□

Index

Immunisation

Immunisation

Live vaccines, 5, 8–10, 17
  BCG, 87–9
  influenza, 104–5
  measles, 66, 68
  mumps, 120
  oral poliovaccine (OPV), 55, 59–61
  rubella, 76–7
  smallpox, 46–7
  yellow fever, 113
Lymphangitis after BCG vaccination, 89–90
Lymphoma, smallpox vaccination contraindication, 17, 50

Mantoux (intradermal) tuberculin test, 83–4
Maternally transmitted antibodies, 13, 44, 69, 126, 133, 134
Measles
  antibacterial drug treatment, 67
  complications
    encephalitis, otitis media, respiratory, 67
  immunisation, 67–73
    and tuberculosis, 73
    in developing countries, 143–4
    natural infection, 4
    with human normal immunoglobulin, 132–3
  mortality rate, 66–7, 70–1
    socioeconomic factors, 1
  outbreak control, 71
  vaccine, 5, 66, 68–9
    killed, 69
    live, 68
    'vaccine disease', 68
  virus, haemagglutinin fraction, 69
Measles–rubella vaccine, 79
Meningitis in mumps, 3, 119
Meningoencephalitis in mumps, 3, 119
Mortality rates
  diphtheria, 18–20, 21–2
  infectious diseases, pre-immunisation era, 2
  measles, 66–7, 70–1
  poliomyelitis, 54, 58
  smallpox, 43–6
  tetanus, 26–7
  tuberculosis, 80–1
  whooping cough, 33, 35–40
  yellow fever, 111–13
Mosquito control in yellow fever, 1, 111
Mumps
  immunisation, 3, 120
  meningitis in, 3, 119
  meningoencephalitis in, 3, 119
  orchitis, 3, 119–20
  pancreatitis, 3, 119

Mycobacterium tuberculosis, attenuated strain, 5

Nephrotic syndrome after measles vaccination, 72
Neuraminidase antigen, influenza, 97–9
Notifications
  in developing countries, 139–40
  of tuberculosis, 81–3

OPV, *see* Oral poliovirus vaccine
Oral poliovirus vaccine (OPV), 55, 59–64
Orchitis, mumps, 3, 119–20
Otitis media complications in measles, 67

Pancreatitis, mumps, 3, 119
Paralysis, infantile, *see* Poliomyelitis
Passive immunisation, 6–7, 126–38, *for specific diseases, see under* Immunisation procedures
Penicillin-free poliovirus vaccine, 58
Plague immunisation, 3, 118
Poliomyelitis
  herd immunity, 58
  immunisation, 11–13, 56–65
    for travel, 117
    in developing countries, 142–3
    natural infection, 4
    outbreak control, 61
    with human normal immunoglobulin, 135
  mortality rate, 54, 58
Polioviruses, 55
Poliovirus vaccines, 5, 9, 55–64
  inactivated (IPV), 55–9
  live attenuated oral (OPV), 55, 59–64
Potentiation of whooping cough by secondary virus infection, 32
Pregnancy
  effect of rubella infection, 74–6
  effect of rubella vaccine, 77–8, 79
  vaccination contraindication
    influenza, 103
    live virus vaccines, 17, 50, 59, 64–5
Psittacosis control, 1

Quadruple vaccine, *see* Dip/tet/pert/polio vaccine
Quintiple vaccine, *see* Dip/tet/pert-/polio/measles vaccine

RA 27/3 rubella virus vaccine, 76–7
Rabies
  antirabies immunoglobulin, 138